# Praise for Rachel Hill's
# Invisible Hypothyroidism

*"After reading Rachel Hill's book, thyroid patients will realize that even though it may seem that their disease isolates them, they are truly never alone."*
— The National Academy of Hypothyroidism

*"Rachel Hill's book guides patients through the many complexities of thyroid hormone health. She helps to provide patients with a roadmap which includes a whole section dedicated to those most important on our journey... Our support network of family and friends with tips on how they can support us. A great read for patients and those who love us."*
- ThyroidChange

*"Rachel Hill's new book "Be Your Own Thyroid Advocate: When You're Sick and Tired of Being Sick and Tired" is a wealth of information about Hashimoto's disease and hypothyroidism. Rachel writes with great passion about her own experience dealing with a thyroid problem that everyone struggling would benefit to read. I especially liked all of the great thyroid resources that Rachel provides. I highly recommend this book to anyone who is suffering from a thyroid disorder and would like to get well."*
— Dr Nikolas Hedberg author of The Complete Thyroid Health and Diet Guide

# Be Your Own Thyroid Advocate

## When You're Sick and Tired of Being Sick and Tired

### Second Edition

RACHEL HILL

# Dedication

To my husband Adam, who has been with me through the whole thyroid journey. I love you with all my heart and couldn't have gotten through everything life has thrown at me without you. Including all this thyroid stuff! My biggest fan. I love you.

## and

To The Thyroid Family, who really uphold what 'family' means; we're there for each other on the good days *and* the not-so-good days. We share the successes *and* struggles. We empower each other to find better health and know that it is indeed out there. I've made great friends with many of you and you were the first to suggest I write a book. My first book is also for you. I hope it lives up to your expectations. Not forgetting the current Thyroid Family administrators and moderators at the time of writing the first edition; Margaret Butler, Elizabeth Waggott, Hedi van Meurs, Lynne Smelt, Joy Rae and Kay Williams, who help me to maintain this online support group of thousands of thyroid patients worldwide. Thank you too. These women give up (a lot of) their own personal time to answer questions, educate and empower others so that we can drive The Invisible Hypothyroidism's message of being your own thyroid advocate further. The number of patients they will have helped is immense.

# Acknowledgements

Adam, my now-husband, who I've been with since I was just sixteen years old and still healthy! You've seen all my declines and improvements in health over the years and you've been more supportive than I could ever have asked for. You encouraged me to blog about my experiences and put it in a book. So, this book certainly wouldn't have happened without you. Especially without your countless hours helping me technically put this book together and getting it published. Thank you also for all the evenings you've spent addressing the technical magic behind my website and more, and for always encouraging me to develop in my work.

The thyroid patients around the world who very kindly read an early copy of this book and provided me with feedback on content. You helped to ensure I delivered what people were wanting in this book.

Louise Champion, a fellow thyroid patient who proofread and provided me with a detailed list of suggested edits.

Ahmad Shoma, who created the illustration of myself on the cover of this book.

Most importantly, this book or any of The Invisible Hypothyroidism's work would not have been possible without all the thyroid patients worldwide who have shared their experiences with me, follow my work, support my work and help me develop. Many of them requested a book and I'm pleased to say it's finally here!

# Disclaimer

This book is compiled to provide information and education on health. It contains information that is intended to help the reader become a better-informed consumer of healthcare. Its publication is not intended to replace the relationship with your doctor or any other medical professional and their guidance. Neither the publisher, author, or anyone involved with making this book, mentioned or quoted in the book, takes responsibility for any consequences of any treatment, actions or application of any method by any person reading or following the information contained in this book.

Therefore it is recommended that you consult with your physician regarding any drugs, supplements, diet changes or other treatments and therapies that may be beneficial to you. This book is not intended as a substitute for the medical advice of a doctor. The reader should regularly consult a physician in matters relating to their health.

Every effort has been made to ensure that this book is as complete and accurate as possible, however, there may be mistakes, both typographical and in content. This book contains information that should be assumed current only up to the printing date. This book should only be used as a guide and not to replace your relationship with your doctor.

Although the author has made every effort to ensure that the information in this book was correct at time of printing, the author does not assume and hereby disclaims any liability or responsibility to any party for any loss, damage, or disruption caused by errors or omissions, whether such errors or omissions result from negligence, accident, or any other cause.

# About the Author

Rachel Hill, creator of The Invisible Hypothyroidism and nominee of eight 2019 WEGO Health Awards, lives in England with her husband Adam. She is a highly ranked and award-winning writer appearing in top thyroid resource lists, as a trusted and valuable contributor to the thyroid community.

As well as a passionate thyroid patient advocate, Rachel is a pretty regular human being. She loves anything vintage and retro, experiencing new cultures and food, being on the beach, walking and exploring and is often consumed by wanderlust. Usually the 'mum' in her friendship groups, she's often found organising themed parties with no theme being too wacky, accompanied by mandatory costumes.

To keep up to date on thyroid news, information and Rachel's personal journey, please visit her website at TheInvisibleHypothyroidism.com, follow her on her social media accounts (Facebook, Instagram, Twitter) or sign up to her newsletter, where you will find she's pored countless hours in to providing as much information for thyroid patients as possible.

*"I want to inspire and reassure people. I want to give those who really need it, hope. I want to reach someone and have them think 'because of you, I didn't give up.'*

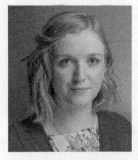

*That's what drives me."*

# Contents

# Preface

*"Perhaps the butterfly is proof that you can go through a great deal of darkness yet become something so beautiful." - Unknown*

Firstly, welcome to my first book.

I'm kind of new to this, I won't lie, but what I hope to have achieved here is a book that resonates with many people around the world. Those with hypothyroidism, those who suspect they have it and then the friends and family of those very people.

First and foremost, I want you to feel reassured that you are **not** alone with thyroid disease. If you're struggling with your thyroid condition right now, then know that I've been there - I've been depressed, fed up, questioned whether it was all in my head and I've felt as if no one on this planet understood what I was going through. Heck, *I* don't even understand my own body some days. But let me tell you: there are thousands of people worldwide who are going through what you are. The confusion, the frustration, the grief for the old you and everything else that tends to come with hypothyroidism. The fatigue, the brain fog, the muscle aches and the *"why me?"*

To the friends and family of those with thyroid disease, I hope to reach you too. I hope to not only open your eyes as to what exactly we experience as thyroid patients, but to also guide you in what you can do to support and help us.

Thank you for being here.

**I'm not a doctor, but another thyroid patient, who got sick and tired of being sick and tired.**

I am one of the many faces of thyroid disease. I am a thyroid advocate for myself but also the many other patients worldwide. Being a thyroid patient who advocates every day for better understanding, knowledge, treatment and awareness, means I have the best experience possible to do the job. I am a Hashimoto's warrior. I am a thyroid advocate and writer. I am passionate about helping those with hypothyroidism and giving them a voice. Because we *need* a voice.

Thyroid disease affects so many people (The World Health Organization estimates that it affects 750 million people in the world[1]) and this could literally be anyone, of all ages, ethnicities, genders, shapes and backgrounds. This is why we need adequate testing and treatment for all. I believe in each patient getting the right treatment *for them*. We're all individuals after all, and this one-size-fits-all approach that so many medical professionals apply is leaving many people unwell. Even if they refuse to acknowledge it.

I began my advocacy journey when I started writing my experiences in the form of a blog, which was yet to go live, in December 2015. I began writing diary entries on Wordpress.com and by March 2016 felt comfortable to finally publish what I had written so far, for others to see. I clicked 'publish' and took a deep breath.

This was the birth of The Invisible Hypothyroidism, my blog. I soon felt overwhelmed by the response; other people confirming that they too had experienced the same struggles in diagnosis and treatment of their hypothyroidism.

People expressing their gratitude for my blog reassuring them that they were not alone in their struggles. People thanking me for educating and empowering them. I was pleased that opening up about something so personal to me was proving to be beneficial to others straight away. It's all I could have hoped for.

But I didn't stop there.

As well as writing about my personal experiences of both my physical and mental health struggles on TheInvisibleHypothyroidism.com, I also began writing informative articles based on research, studies, science and other reputable sites and blogs, too. I also began writing articles for The Mighty, producing posts about the lesser known issues and struggles of living with hypothyroidism, such as poor mental health and everything else that often comes with it. I worked hard to reach as many thyroid patients around the world as possible, by spreading the word about my online Support Group 'The Thyroid Family' and having my articles and blogs shared and republished across many other sites and publications.

I've written for The National Academy of Hypothyroidism and ThyroidChange, which, when they first reached out to me, blew my mind. I have worked with the BBC, Yahoo, Thyroid Refresh, The NAH, ThyroidChange, Dr Nikolas Hedberg, MSN and Nutritionist Emily Kyle on a Thyroid Cookbook, and more (the cookbook is listed at the back of this book).

The Invisible Hypothyroidism's work is supported by The National Academy of Hypothyroidism as they Awarded me with 'One Of The Top Thyroid Blogs You

Need to Read' and they also cited me as one of the best thyroid advocates doing their part to raise thyroid awareness. I also have the support of ThyroidChange, Dr Nikolas Hedberg, Jeffrey Dach MD, Stop The Thyroid Madness and more, who have all included The Invisible Hypothyroidism in their thyroid patient resource lists. This very book *Be Your Own Thyroid Advocate* has been cited in HealthRising.org's article on the use of T3 thyroid medications in Chronic Fatigue Syndrome.

In 2019, I was nominated for eight WEGO Health Awards, The Best Personal Development Blog award at the Annual Bloggers Bash Awards, and I have been included in the Top 10 for the Top Hypothyroidism Websites List and Top Thyroid Websites List.

The Invisible Hypothyroidism gets involved in lots of other good thyroid stuff too that is forever evolving, and this is very exciting. I am frequently interviewed for articles and podcasts, feature in research projects, publications, documentaries and more. I speak very openly about thyroid disease in all work that I do and on all my social media accounts. I have also released a book for our loved ones, *You, Me and Hypothyroidism: When Someone You Love Has Hypothyroidism,* in order to help those around us to understand what the thyroid patient in their life experiences. In 2019, I also launched Thoughtful Thyroid, which hosts online courses for thyroid patients to take, that help them to achieve better health too.

At the core of my work, I hold raising awareness of hypothyroidism and helping other thyroid patients, as the key purpose and it is what gets me out of bed in the morning and helps me sleep at night; knowing I have made a difference to someone's life that day.

You see, when I say that I am passionate about giving thyroid patients a voice, reaching and helping as many as possible and spreading general awareness so that people become more aware of the symptoms and struggles of the disease, I *really* do mean it. And writing a book is my next step in doing that. I hope it will reach those who perhaps don't have a computer or follow online blogs and websites for information and so are disadvantaged somewhat in improving their thyroid health. I hope it will reach family members of thyroid patients who are desperately needing their support. I hope it shines more light on the condition and creates even more room to discuss the difficulties, struggles and issues surrounding the condition. I hope it cements all the work I have done so far in the *internet* world.

I have always been a kind-hearted, compassionate and emotional person and I have always had this innate need to help other people. I've considered careers in caring, nursing and even as an agony aunt, but none of them were quite right and it seems I have found my path now as an advocate for the many thyroid warriors worldwide.

Writing, advocating and representing hypothyroid patients is what I live for. It's my passion. It keeps me going on dark days of living with this disease.

Now, I had so much that I wanted to cover in this book, my first book, having written around four hundred articles and blogs online to date. But alas, that would have meant hundreds of chapters! I do hope that *Be Your Own Thyroid Advocate: When You're Sick and Tired of Being Sick and Tired* is at least an introduction and solid basis. And if you're not sick of me by the end of this book, lots more material and resources can be found in my online courses, on my website and social media platforms too. Or maybe one day, I'll put together another book to expand on this one. Who knows!

Keeping authenticity and raw honesty behind my work, I won't ever lie about my own experiences; I really have struggled to come to terms with living with a chronic illness. In fact, I still grieve for my old self on tough thyroid days, but what I *can* do is turn a negative experience into something useful and positive.

As my friend Svenja once said to me:

*"You've taken something that could have been devastating and turned it into a positive by helping other people."*

And I think that's what I was put on this Earth to do.

Rachel, The Invisible Hypothyroidism

# Introduction

*"I am spending the rest of my life making other people feel less lost." - Rachel Hill, The Invisible Hypothyroidism*

*Be Your Own Thyroid Advocate: When You're Sick and Tired of Being Sick and Tired* is, I hope, a uniquely honest and authentic recounting of my own personal journey back to good health with hypothyroidism and Hashimoto's disease, including all the ups and downs, the successes and brick walls I experienced and a reassurance that you are not alone in your own thyroid journey. It remains true to myself and my work, not only in the personal experiences shared, but also the *way* in which I have written about them. This book is written in my usual style and that which I am known for and have been praised for in the online world and community. It may seem a little different to other thyroid books to begin with, but I hope my own flair and voice helps to reaffirm that these experiences are from a real person.

As well as my own story recounted throughout the book, I have also included the crucial information I learnt along the way, which helped me back to good health. A lot of the information shared with you here is from a functional medicine viewpoint so it's worth noting that conventional medicine doctors may well not follow it all. This is why being your *own* healthcare advocate is so important. Those who get better from becoming ill with thyroid disease are often those who take responsibility.

The purpose of this book is to arm *you*, the thyroid patient or loved one of a thyroid patient, who is still unwell despite being on thyroid medication, with the knowledge and mindset needed to regain and reinstate a good quality of life. Because believe it or not - it can be achieved.

There are some thyroid patients who of course do absolutely fine on standard thyroid medication such as Levothyroxine and Synthroid, but the purpose of my book is to let those who do not, know that there are other options out there that could help them instead.

I still see a regular GP on the NHS here in England who is supportive of my current non-conventional thyroid medication and has been of great help to me in managing my health, so I don't completely reject traditional medical practises; I am just providing a different light and the alternatives that I know others will benefit to know of. Mainstream or conventional medicine is great in so many ways and for many other health conditions, but in my experience it can let some people with thyroid disease down.

When I was reading various books, websites and work by thyroid doctors and advocates whilst very ill myself, I oftentimes found it hard to absorb a lot of it and even understand some of the phrasing or detail, so I hope to have formed a book that is easy to understand, follow and then use in your own thyroid journey. Especially for those of us who experience thyroid brain fog! I wanted to create an easy to follow yet informative book that sounds as if it's coming from a friend, as I found that information on some websites and books were written quite scarily and negatively or included a lot of jargon we quite honestly don't need to know as thyroid patients. We just need the important bits.

You may ask what my qualifications are to have written this book, and whilst I'm not a doctor, I have various qualifications and certificates (and am often studying for more) in many subjects and topics that help my mission.

Perhaps the most relevant are in Diet and Nutrition, Reflexology and Life Coaching, which are useful in my role as a thyroid advocate. But what makes me best qualified is being an extremely experienced thyroid patient expert myself. It enables me to speak for thyroid patients around the globe who are still unwell and also share what has (and hasn't) helped us. Well-recognised as a valuable contributor to the thyroid community, my work is award-winning and I am always working with experts in the thyroid disease field, to change and improve the lives of thyroid patients.

As many other thyroid patients will relate, having hypothyroidism and Hashimoto's left me sick and tired of being sick and tired, and as a result I soon became extremely well-read in literature regarding thyroid disease and the intricacies involved when treating and managing an individual with it. And so, with a thirst to absorb as much as I could about this little butterfly shaped gland in my neck, I started to share everything I had learnt and built relationships with key figures in the field. As a thyroid patient who has had to learn all the ins and outs of the condition in order to get herself better, I have been able to filter the best information and locate the tools hypothyroid patients needs to regain good health once more.

I do not dislike or hate doctors so please don't interpret my personal story as that. Despite my various negative encounters with medical professionals which are shared in this book, my current doctors are great. It's just that unfortunately, I have experienced a fair few who were not helpful and that is sadly just part of my journey that lead me to where I am today. Giving completeness in my writing is very important to me.

## Make Sure You're Not Hindering Your Recovery

The message behind all my work and including this book, is to be your own thyroid advocate. But what does this mean?

Let me start by saying that I write as someone who has been in a place of poor mental health, horrendous physical health, high stress, massive frustration, bitterness and a victim mentality.

Just like many of you with the same health conditions, I too went through life for a while feeling angry, frustrated and sick and tired of being sick and tired. I felt like there were no options to improve my health and situation, and so I felt hopeless. My depression and anxiety led me to the point of being suicidal as my life fell apart all around me and I felt I had no control. *It was all so unfair.* But what I eventually realised, was that by being bitter and angry, I was only making my situation worse. I was *hindering* my health. And how pointless is it to make your bad situation even worse?

So, after standing by for long enough, I had to decide to take charge and responsibility (because let's face it, often no one else takes responsibility for our thyroid health *for* us) and decide that it was *on me* to improve my situation. I began advocating for my health.

Whether you manage to have your current doctor take some of the information presented here on board, seek out a different type of doctor or decide to make a start on implementing small changes that can lead to big improvements yourself, the key is to become your own thyroid advocate. By this, I mean becoming more active in your own healthcare, understanding what's going on i.e. with test results and medication options, and researching and reading up to empower yourself with crucial knowledge.

**Here's the wakeup call you may need: you're not going to move forward without taking personal responsibility for this.**

I eventually realised this myself.

Within a few months of taking things back in to my own hands and taking back control, I was free of depression and my anxiety was much improved. I was back in work and my home life and social life were great once again. But there's no magic way to snap your fingers and have it all sorted out and even the best medical professional won't be able to help you without you adjusting your mindset, which I know can be hard with mental health difficulties such as depression. But one step at a time and you *will* get there.

You may be reading this and thinking that changing your mindset isn't relevant to your situation. It could well be the case that you've already assumed this responsibility but if you haven't then that's OK too. We all come to realise how important our mindset is in our own time. But as time goes on and thyroid patients don't realise that they need to embrace being an active participant in their own healthcare, they end up losing more time to this disease and become increasingly unhappy. And that's heart-breaking because it really doesn't have to be that way. You *can* live a good quality life with hypothyroidism and Hashimoto's. Many of us are doing this!

But first, you need to break free of victim mentality and instead embrace advocating for yourself. If you're guilty of this.

Many thyroid patients are starting their journey back to good health through becoming their own thyroid advocate every single day. Don't delay yours any longer.

# Chapter 1: What on Earth Is Wrong with Me?!

*"I'd like a refund on my body please. It's expensive to run and full of defects." - Unknown*

How much am I willing to bet that getting an eventual diagnosis of hypothyroidism wasn't just difficult for me, but for others, too?

I guess you could say that symptoms of a thyroid problem started for me at just sixteen years old. After having a bout of swine flu (yep, I was unfortunately affected, you'll soon gather that I don't have much luck), I was left with a recurring ache in my legs, which would plague me a few times a week in the evenings. The only cause I was sure of was that it happened on days I walked or exercised more than usual, but doctors had no clue what caused it apart from the swine flu and I was told that it was *just a lingering effect'* of that. Even after it had well passed.

But even before that unfortunate run in with a crazy strain of flu, I had tell-tale signs of someone who was eventually going to develop autoimmune hypothyroidism anyway. From a young age, I lacked energy, to the point that people frequently called me lazy and assumed I just hated moving off the sofa. Until I was eighteen years old, I didn't realise that it wasn't normal to only be going for bowel movements once or twice a week and had even gone one or two weeks between going before. My periods have always been a nightmare, from starting them at age twelve I experienced irregular cycles and incredibly painful and heavy periods that often had me soaking through the heaviest sanitary towel every half an hour. I'd come home from school needing to change my clothes from leaking horrendously, every single month. And don't even get me started on the size of the blood clots. It was nothing short of horrendous. I knew it wasn't right, even from a young age; I knew my *body* wasn't right.

So yes, I was likely always going to trigger Hashimoto's (the autoimmune condition which causes over 90% of hypothyroid cases[2]). The signs were there. Contracting swine flu just brought it that bit closer to going full blown earlier on in life.

But another round of flu hit me at seventeen years old, which was so bad I ended up in hospital with dehydration and then, when the doctors couldn't help, I developed pneumonia and ended up in intensive care. I'm told by Adam, my now-husband, that I could have died and at one point, they weren't sure if I was going to make it. Truth be told, I barely remember any of it myself. I remember the first few days after being admitted to the ward and then the sudden panic when I couldn't breathe properly, but apart from that, I only have a few foggy memories of spending my eighteenth birthday on life support and some nurses trying to ram a feeding tube down my throat without consent. I've since avoided going back to hospital wherever possible. Unsurprisingly!

Another round of flu and then pneumonia attacking my body at just seventeen years old, less than two years after the swine flu, was too much for me to take and I was soon left anaemic and with around 80% of my hair having fallen out.

In between the two bouts of flu, I experienced some major life stresses and trauma, which made me particularly vulnerable to catching the second round of crazy flu. At seventeen, my stable family home was broken up and I moved around in terms of where I lived, was put under a ridiculous amount of stress for someone of such a young age and soon became depressed and anxiety ridden. I've always been a worrier but let me tell you, anxiety is very different. I wasn't sleeping right, had diarrhoea constantly, wasn't eating well and was always on high alert for everything. I know now that my adrenal glands were under a lot of pressure at this point and the stress I was going through, at no fault of my own, was another huge trigger for the Hashimoto's. It helped to wear down my immune system and so by the time I contracted the flu yet again, there wasn't much of a chance for me to fight it off.

In just a couple of years, my body had gone through so much emotional, mental and physical stress, that Hashimoto's was well under way and thriving in the environment created. I'd hammered a lot of triggers in a short space of time, unknowingly. From this point on, it became a running joke that I was always sickly, catching anything going around, always full of a cold and at the doctor's office for something or other. It's true. During these five years or so leading up to my eventual diagnosis, I was back at the doctor's most months, complaining of a new frustrating symptom, building up over twenty separate symptoms with no reason or cause for them.

They included: fatigue, muscle and joint aches and pains, brain fog, confusion, long recovery times, brittle hair and nails, sensitivity to cold (cold hands and feet), poor appetite, inability to lose weight, slow in movement, thoughts and speech, hoarse voice, thinned eyebrows, constipation, acid reflux, migraines, anxiety, dry and tight skin, heavy periods, hot flashes, body heaviness, depression, numbness in limbs, weight gain, very emotional all the time, excessive wind, leg cramping, menstrual spotting, restless legs, constantly itchy and sore scalp and always worsening fatigue.

No one ever had an answer for me, especially as I was so young. I was given various medications that didn't help, yet all these seemingly unrelated annoyances were piling up and they were bugging me. I was growing increasingly concerned but told myself *"I'm just being a hypochondriac. The doctor's know what they're doing,"* and kept brushing the niggling feeling in the pit of my stomach away.

*Did the doctors really know best, though?* It wasn't until I went back again complaining of ongoing fatigue still, aged 20 by this time, that they finally thought to check my thyroid levels. In fact, they'd only ever checked my iron before this. Now I was finally being checked for low thyroid, glandular fever, Vitamin D, Iron, Ferritin, B12, diabetes and more. It was this particular GPs last day at work before retiring and so I sometimes wonder if I just caught her on a good day, where she was willing to go all out on the tests because she was retiring an hour later anyway. Had I seen someone else, would I have been waiting even longer for a diagnosis?

As I sat in that office and she said *"I'm going to test you for glandular fever, low iron and an underactive thyroid gland as well as some other things",* this strange moment of realisation came over me. I remember my mum mentioning the phrase 'underactive thyroid gland' in my childhood. I was no longer in contact with any of my biological family by this point, so I couldn't ask them, but I'm sure she wasn't diagnosed with an underactive thyroid. I knew she was on iron supplements at times but I'd have known if she was on thyroid medication, surely? In fact, she was hardly ever at the doctors, so then why did it sound so familiar?

I can only assume that my mum would mention it from time to time with examples such as *"If she's gained weight, has she been checked for a gland problem?"* and *"Being tired all the time could be a thyroid problem."* due to having knowledge of *someone* in the family with hypothyroidism. Which would make sense since it is often hereditary.

But it's still a mystery to me. I am pretty certain that my mum and possibly one or two other family members have hypothyroidism as well and I wonder if they've been tested or diagnosed since I was last in touch.

Whilst waiting for my thyroid test results to come back, I googled 'thyroid problem' and all the related phrases to unearth why it sounded so familiar to me. And a light bulb went on as I read other patient experiences on the NHS website. Comments left explained how people were bed-bound with the fatigue, had to give up their job from the brain fog and mental degeneration and were depressed and feeling hopeless, even after starting thyroid medication. Leg cramps, migraines, acid reflux, fatigue, depression… they were all there. As a sudden wave of shock came over me, I felt stuck to the bed I was sitting in. My body frozen like stone; everything suddenly pieced together. All the symptoms I had been going back to the doctor's with, the aching legs and ill health, all the pieces of this jigsaw puzzle I never realised were connected, slotted together. It was a bizarre moment. An awakening if you will, five years in the making.

And sure enough, the test results came back a few days later to confirm Hashimoto's Thyroiditis, with an off the charts TPOAB result of greater than 1300, and 'borderline' hypothyroidism.

## What is Hypothyroidism?

Hypothyroidism, also called an underactive thyroid or thyroid disease, is a condition where the thyroid gland, located at the front of your neck, does not create enough thyroid hormone. The five hormones a healthy thyroid produces are: T1, T2, T3, T4 and Calcitonin, with the most important being T3 and T4; T3 the most active.

These hormones are needed for every process, every cell and every function in the body, so when they go wrong i.e. are too low, a lot of other stuff goes wrong too.

This can include:

- Metabolic function
- Sensitivity to heat and cold intolerance
- Muscle/joint aches and pains, cramps and weakness
- Fatigue
- Adrenal problems
- Vitamin deficiencies
- Weight gain and inability to lose weight
- Constipation and/or wind often
- Depression, anxiety and other mental health difficulties
- Slow movements, speech and thoughts
- Itchy and sore scalp
- Poor appetite
- Dry and tight feeling skin
- Brittle hair and nails

- Loss of libido (sex drive)
- Pain, numbness and a tingling sensation in the hand and fingers (carpal tunnel syndrome)
- Numbness in limbs
- Period problems
- Brain fog/confusion/memory problems
- Migraines
- Hoarse voice
- A puffy-looking face
- Thinned or partly missing eyebrows
- A slow heart rate or one that increases more so than a healthy person's, after physical activity (e.g. after walking up the stairs or emptying the washing machine)
- Hearing loss
- Poor stamina
- Feeling weak
- The need to nap more than others
- Long recovery period after any activity
- Inability to exercise, or withstand certain exercises
- Diagnosis of Chronic Fatigue Syndrome
- Being overly emotional
- Poor circulation
- High or rising cholesterol
- Acid reflux
- IBS
- Hair loss

- Easy bruising
- Swollen legs that impede walking
- Shin splints
- Difficulty standing on feet
- Fertility issues

Many people find that they have their own combination of this long list of symptoms or even experience something not shown here. In fact, this list is by no means exhaustive; I'm always hearing about new symptoms. As thyroid hormone is required for every cell and every function in the body, when we don't have enough of them, the effects are far reaching.

The main purpose of thyroid hormone is to ensure that the metabolism is running properly with the metabolism's job being to produce heat and fuel. Heat to keep us warm and fuel to give us energy. Now, if we don't have enough of those thyroid hormones, our metabolism won't work properly and so can't provide us with adequate heat and fuel. Therefore, people with an underactive thyroid (hypothyroidism) have a slow metabolism, so will have symptoms associated with a slow metabolism, such as cold intolerance (from the lack of heat made) and extreme tiredness and weight gain (from the lack of calories burned to make energy).

Hypothyroidism affects its hosts differently, as some people report taking their medication each day and feeling fine, whereas other patients report that their medication does not help them, or that it did at one time, but not anymore.

Ultimately, once thyroid levels are optimal and the thyroid condition is being optimally addressed, most symptoms should start to disappear, but support for other possible problems like vitamin deficiencies and adrenal dysfunction for example, will need to be in place until they recover, too.

However, as you're going to learn in this book, it's often not as simple as taking a thyroid pill once a day and being able to run a marathon the next. Hypothyroidism is often mistaken for being an easy to treat condition, but it really isn't for many people.

## What is 'Borderline' or 'Subclinical' Hypothyroidism?

A someone who was diagnosed with a 'borderline underactive thyroid', I always wince at the phrase. Although my TSH test may have been borderline, my symptoms certainly were not. In fact, I was told, when at a point of barely functioning anymore, to come back in a few months' time for a repeat thyroid test to be reviewed again because I wasn't yet 'bad enough' to receive treatment. To no surprise, when I returned a few months later, I was feeling absolutely dreadful. And I looked absolutely dreadful! By the time of the repeat test, my results were only slightly worse and still 'mildly' hypothyroid, but I was started on Levothyroxine to see if it helped because I complained about my symptoms so loudly.

In my opinion, I feel that the term 'borderline hypothyroid' or 'subclinical hypothyroidism' used when a doctor refuses treatment, is them acknowledging that your thyroid isn't performing well, but not yet bad enough to receive medication. It's like a limbo stage and I really feel that it's disgusting to leave people there, without any further support or guidance on their health. Some stay in this limbo for years, going back to the doctor numerous times only to be told they're still 'borderline' and refused any further help.

The problem is that many doctors just go by the TSH test when testing thyroid function, which doesn't give us the full picture, and while TSH may only be 'mildly' bad, Free T3 and Free T4 levels can be much lower, leading to symptoms of hypothyroidism. These are also the actual thyroid hormone levels, with TSH being a pituitary hormone. Being optimal in thyroid hormone levels can make all the difference for a lot of people, but subclinical or borderline hypothyroidism leaves many people with low levels in Free T3 and Free T4, causing ongoing symptoms because they are actually hypothyroid. And it's important to keep in mind that test ranges differ from lab to lab and country to country. The inconsistency on what constitutes for 'borderline' hypothyroidism is shocking.

Not only is going by TSH alone inaccurate in diagnosing and treating hypothyroidism, but subjecting everyone to outdated ranges is problematic since many of us see the effects of a high TSH differently. For example, the range my doctor used at the beginning was I believe 0.5-10, and I felt very ill at 9, which is just within range; borderline. I've heard some people get to a TSH of 4, 50 or even 100 before feeling unwell, therefore, we should be treated individually.

A TSH of 0.5-2 is recommended under many guidelines these days, so even if you're classed as borderline with a TSH reading of 6 on a 0.5-5 range, then this can be causing you a lot of symptoms. The same goes for a Free T4 of 11 when the range is 10-20, for example. These wide ranges do not take in to account where each individual feels best and so doctors would be helping us more if they worked to find this sweet spot for each patient instead of just looking to see if we fall within range. We're individuals and deserve to be treated as such, after all.

Since most of us didn't have our TSH, Free T3 and Free T4 levels tested when our thyroid function was good, we don't know our individual optimal levels, so we must work to find these.

If your doctor has said you're borderline or subclinically hypothyroid and refuses to look any further in to treatment options, despite you feel unwell, then I strongly suggest you get another doctor's opinion, and possibly another, until you find someone who will look at addressing your symptoms, even if you're 'only borderline' hypothyroid. You should also have a retest of any borderline TSH, Free T3 or Free T4 readings to see if they have become better or worse. They can occasionally get better, but for many, they get progressively worse.

It is also worth noting that Hashimoto's, the autoimmune disease behind most hypothyroidism cases, can cause TSH levels to move up and down. This is due to thyroid cells being damaged or destroyed from Hashimoto's disease and releasing their stored thyroid hormone into the bloodstream, which can make thyroid hormone levels look higher temporarily. So, if you still feel unwell and have blood test results that seem to get better and worse again, it's a possibility that you have Hashimoto's, which definitely needs confirming.

## Chapter Recap:

- Hypothyroidism often develops slowly over time with symptoms that increase to match.

- Hashimoto's, the leading cause of hypothyroidism, is 'triggered' and being able to pinpoint what triggered yours can be helpful in understanding how to manage your health in future.

- Borderline or subclinical hypothyroidism can still cause a lot of symptoms and should be monitored closely and regularly, and if suitable, addressed with medication or other treatment.

# Chapter 2: My Eventual Diagnosis

*"Just as the caterpillar thought its life was over, it grew wings and began to fly." - Unknown*

As I heard my suspicions confirmed by the doctor, who gave me the diagnosis of autoimmune 'subclinical' hypothyroidism so casually, I actually felt relieved. I finally had an answer. It was finally confirmed that *I wasn't mad and it wasn't all in my head, after all these years.*

He signed a prescription for Levothyroxine, the standard T4-only medication for hypothyroidism, and thrust it into my hands as I took a huge sigh of relief. He even told me that here in the UK, we get prescriptions for thyroid medication for free. *That's great,* I thought. *An added bonus.*

Aged twenty-one, I left that doctor's office and happily took my prescription to be filled at the nearest pharmacy, but as I took a seat and waited for it, I suddenly began to fill with dread. I was beginning a medication that I would now be on *for life* and I was still so young. The doctor hadn't really explained to me what the antibodies meant, what my thyroid was or what my prognosis was going forward, I was just given a medication that I was told would fix my symptoms and make everything well again. Then I was sent on my way.

This isn't unusual for thyroid patients. I hear all the time from people who were told to *"just take this pill once a day and you'll be fine."* They've been told they have a condition they'll have for life and then sent out the door to deal with it themselves. Then when they start looking online for information, doctors get angry that they

35

shouldn't be *'reading that rubbish on the world wide web'* in the absence of their help.

As I waited for my prescription, following the diagnosis just minutes earlier, I began to feel very daunted by the whole idea and I soon found myself going through a whirlwind of emotion - fear, confusion, frustration, anger, sadness, relief and grief. Fear for what else was to come; I'd already experienced so many horrible effects of hypothyroidism. Confusion about what exactly was *wrong* with me. Frustration regarding why it had taken so long to finally get to the bottom of my five yearlong battle. Anger because I didn't understand *why* it was me having to go through this at a young age. Sadness for the many aspects of my life affected - work, social, personal. Relief for finally having an answer. And the big one, grief. Grief for the path I thought I was going to have in life, aged twenty-one with my life ahead of me, but feeling as if it was now going to be forever different, the image of my future forever changed and impossible to get back.

People rarely speak about the grief you go through when diagnosed with a life-altering illness, but it can be huge. The world suddenly looks very different. Darker, even.

You see, for me, receiving that diagnosis of a lifelong, chronic health condition seemed to change everything. It wasn't anaemia that I could recover from within a few months and then bounce back to how I was before. Being diagnosed with autoimmune hypothyroidism felt like a life sentence. I had read the experiences of other thyroid patients online, whilst I was waiting for the test results to come back, in anticipation of being diagnosed with the same condition and although some found that medication helped, many others never seemed to fully recover. They complained of ongoing heavy fatigue, muscle aches and pains, thinning hair and fertility issues, just to name a few of the many complaints.

Yes, I finally had a reason, a legitimate explanation, for feeling as if I had the flu constantly. For being forgetful and feeling confused. For feeling tired and 'lazy' no matter how much sleep or rest I got. I finally had a reason for struggling for so long and was starting to join the dots in my declining health since I was just sixteen years old.

But it began to dawn on me that I may experience fertility issues one day, that I may struggle to conceive and carry children to full-term and that I will also need a lot of extra help in raising them, due to the effects of hypothyroidism. This may seem crazy and over the top to those who don't understand the full effects of this disease, but failure to properly maintain adequate thyroid levels whilst pregnant can result in complications such as miscarriage, preeclampsia, anaemia, stillbirth and the baby developing congenital hypothyroidism itself. Caring for someone else suddenly seemed really scary when I was now needing a lot of help myself, too.

I realised that I couldn't be as active as I once was and that I needed to compromise on what I *could* do without making myself more ill. I used to walk a lot, run, play badminton and do dance lessons, but my body couldn't keep up anymore, and it was time to reassess. I had to accept that my house wasn't always going to be as clean and tidy as it used to be because I had to learn to prioritise my energy. I had to learn quickly that my body wasn't as strong and capable as it once was and that some days I would be forgetful, achy and fatigued beyond words.

I began to mourn the person I was before I developed hypothyroidism, as well as the life I imagined I would have. Everything seemed like it was going to be different now.

Being so young, at just twenty-one years old, I felt that the life I planned to have - a driven, successful career, a healthy and efficiently run family, an active lifestyle etc. was taken away from me. Not only was I grieving for my life before diagnosis and how this would now change, but I was also grieving for the future I'd planned to have. At twenty-one, I was struggling to keep up with my friends already. I didn't go out partying, rarely drank at all and struggled to maintain in full time work, due to the physical and mental effects of hypothyroidism I had been experiencing. Yet, how was I going to explain this to people? Thyroid problems aren't well understood anyway, but get someone who looks young and somewhat fit to try and explain that they spend most their time in bed unwell and with no quality of life, and people just look at you blankly.

This is where The Spoon Theory came in very useful after my diagnosis. (I have also covered it in more detail in Chapter 11: Dear Friends and Family).

## The Spoon Theory

When people ask me what a Spoonie is and I explain that I have a limited amount of energy that affects my day to day life, so much so that I have to plan my use of energy (spoons), wisely, I often receive a nod of recognition. But I have also been told *"You're too young to have a chronic health condition!"* or *"You won't be really ill for years yet."* Erm. I *do* have a chronic illness. A few, actually. And I *have* been really ill! What has age got to do with it? Does my body care if I'm twenty or eighty? Nope, not at all!

But people generally just don't get it. And that's the beauty of the spoon theory. If you're not familiar with it, let me explain:

Christine Miserandino created the spoon theory[3] to illustrate how many people with a disability or chronic illness must carefully plan their daily activities in order to use their energy wisely, whilst most people with better health or who do not have a disability, do not need to worry about running out of energy for daily tasks. Spoons are the unit of measurement used to track how much energy a person has throughout the day. If you imagine that each activity requires a certain number of spoons, which will only be replaced as the person rests, then if you run out of spoons, you have no choice but to rest until your spoons are replenished. When you live with limited 'spoons', you have to work out what activities you can afford to do each day, so as not to run out of them (energy) and be left exhausted or burnt out.

As those without a disability or chronic illness do not feel the impact of spending spoons for mundane tasks such as bathing and getting dressed, they may not realise the amount of energy used by those who *do* need to plan their energy usage just to get through the day. They do not tend to have a limited amount of energy, as most daily tasks could never come close to exhausting them, unlike some people with hypothyroidism, for example.

The spoon theory is brilliant in helping to explain how we may become tired quicker than others, how we learn to better manage our energy and how, on some days, all we can do is rest. The spoon theory helped my husband and I a lot.

## Dealing with My Diagnosis

Once the initial negative feelings I felt when being diagnosed with autoimmune hypothyroidism began to settle, I started to see more clearly and new emotions came to light. I began to feel hopeful, as researching about my new diagnosis online led me to realise that there was a possibility of a better quality of life. There is *so* much available in books and online to educate ourselves with and become our own advocates (I've included a list of these at the end of this book).

I started to be kinder to myself and shifted blame from me overexerting my body, not pushing doctors enough and struggling to cope with life in general, to the doctors who had failed me and let me down. As I spoke to other thyroid patients and we shared our stories, it became evident that many go undiagnosed for even longer than I did and by the time they *are* diagnosed, they've developed countless other conditions and symptoms, gone through a divorce because of the strain it put on their relationship, lost their job from sickness and not been able to have children as they wished. And I started to become angry.

I became frustrated and shocked that so many people out there were living a life less than they deserved. In fact, a lot aren't even living, they're just existing, and why is that fair? It's not our fault we developed this condition but we're clearly being let down on a massive scale. So many people were complaining that T4-only medications such as Levothyroxine and Synthroid weren't helping, that their doctors were telling them it was all in their heads and that they just couldn't go on anymore. People are actually suicidal and I dread to think of those that may have even taken their lives due to it. I just can't think about it. It's shocking to say the least.

Within a few months of being diagnosed, I had gone through a whirlwind of emotion but now, I was ready to fight. Fight for a better quality of life for myself but also for the many others around the world I was now aware about. The vulnerable and broken down. The many in need of help. I just kept thinking: *After all, why don't we deserve as good a quality of life as the next person?*

One of the first things that was important for me to confirm was whether my hypothyroidism was autoimmune. And indeed, it was. It is estimated that around 90% of hypothyroidism cases are caused by the autoimmune disease Hashimoto's Thyroiditis, or Hashi's for short. This is one thing you absolutely must find out for your own case of thyroid disease as it can affect your treatment and management going forward.

Luckily, I was one of the few who had this confirmed upon diagnosis of hypothyroidism. Knowing I had Hashimoto's meant I needed to look at some other areas of my life in order to make further progress in my health.

And this is number one in my many things I need to share with you, when it comes to getting your health back on the right track too.

## Hashimoto's Thyroiditis: The Most Common Cause for Hypothyroidism

You may be reading this book right now and have no idea that you even have this autoimmune disease. You may have never even been tested, but knowing whether it is the cause for your thyroid problem is beneficial in your treatment and making progress in how you feel.

First off, to know if you have Hashimoto's, you need two tests: TPOAB (Thyroid Peroxidase Antibodies) and TGAB (Thyroglobulin Antibodies). You need both tested preferably, as often just the one test is not accurate enough to be sure. One could have results 'in range', while the other not.

Having Hashimoto's will usually show as TPOAB and TGAB test results being above range, but did you know that you can still have Hashimoto's, without the positive antibodies? Yes, negative antibodies do not necessarily mean that you don't have the autoimmune condition. Because we know that Hashimoto's is responsible for around 90% of those with hypothyroidism, that leaves up to 10% having Hashimoto's but coming back negative on antibody tests. This can be due to a number of reasons, such as antibody numbers moving up and down and catching the lower number when you test, or certain lifestyle interventions such as selenium and Vitamin D supplementation, gluten and dairy free diets all supposedly lowering antibodies in some patients, or your overall immune system being so weak that you do not produce enough of the antibodies, as suggested by Dr Datis Kharrazian.[4]

It is worth knowing that you could see variations in your thyroid antibody and TSH results each time you test though, with them being high one time and low the next, as they swing up and down. This is a common sign of Hashimoto's as ongoing destruction of your thyroid gland causes sudden surges of thyroid hormone to be released into the blood.

It is common for most doctors to refuse to test your thyroid antibodies, though, as they often don't see the importance of knowing whether your hypothyroidism is autoimmune, because for many doctors, they're only going to give you the standard T4-only medication whether you have Hashimoto's or not. But they're wrong, it matters hugely. You could choose to go private to have these tests done if your doctor refuses, or even order them yourself online[5]. I soon learnt that many thyroid patients had turned to doing this and started to myself. It has since been a huge step in recovering my health but also making me feel more empowered about it too.

If your doctor doesn't diagnose you with Hashimoto's when your antibody levels are out of range and TSH still in range, then this is incorrect. As antibodies above range equal Hashimoto's alone. Going by TSH alone for any treatment, diagnosis and management of an underactive thyroid is not ideal anyway, since it is a pituitary hormone, not a thyroid one and doesn't present a full picture. Thyroid hormone levels Free T3 and Free T4 should be checked to gauge how much the Hashimoto's may have affected your thyroid hormone output so far.

## So, what exactly *is* Hashimoto's?

Hashimoto's is an autoimmune disease that causes the body to attack and destroy its own thyroid gland, leading to hypothyroidism as the thyroid begins to dysfunction (lose ability to produce as much thyroid hormone as it should) from the damage caused. As time goes by, if this autoimmune disease is not well controlled, your own body continues to destroy the thyroid, causing a loss of function, which can lead to test results getting gradually worse, meaning further increases in thyroid medication dosage and worsening symptoms.

## What causes Hashimoto's?

It is believed that those of us who develop Hashimoto's, have always carried the genetic makeup to develop it, but then 'switch it on' by triggering it. Triggers for Hashimoto's are widely said to include adrenal fatigue (though it is more accurately referred to as hypothalamic-pituitary axis dysfunction), chronic stress, toxins, poor diet, food sensitivities, viral infections, vitamin deficiencies, EBV, leaky gut, iodine deficiency, use of contraceptive pills, a blow to the immune system such as severe illness or pregnancy, to name just a few.

In my case, I hammered several triggers in a short space of time. By the time I was finally diagnosed, I had been through huge amounts of mental and emotional stress, some particularly nasty illnesses, 'adrenal fatigue', antibiotics, iron anaemia and use of the contraceptive pill.

## What difference does it make if you *do* have Hashimoto's?

Well, it means that you should ideally be looking at calming down the attack on your thyroid gland and lowering those high antibody levels. By doing this, it is believed that the attack against your thyroid is slowed down or even halted, meaning that symptoms disappear and recovery can begin.

Besides just taking thyroid medication, you'll probably need to consider some other things too. It's very much individual, as different people find that different interventions help them to get their health back on track. So, I'm not here to tell you that *you must do this and you must do that*. I am instead presenting you with my findings after a lot of research and then what you do with that information is totally up to you. Be your own advocate; but be proactive.

## Gluten

Most commonly, cutting out gluten from your diet entirely is said to be the most beneficial thing a Hashimoto's patient can do to relieve Hashimoto's symptoms and high antibodies. Research is building up as we speak, which supports this. This is due to gluten triggering the same autoimmune reactions that cause you to have Hashimoto's in the first place, since the cells of your thyroid are similar to the molecular structure of gluten (referred to as molecular mimicry), and it confuses your body, increasing inflammation and antibody levels as an attack on your thyroid is launched, destroying even more thyroid tissue, and so worse hypothyroid symptoms occur.

As a result, many Hashimoto's patients eliminate gluten from their diet, and see good results.

In my opinion, something like this is always worth a trial to see if it works for you, and giving it a few months (at least) will give you a good idea on whether it helps you. You do sadly have to go completely gluten-free (no sneaky 'once a week' glutenous treats or beers) in order for it to work, so don't think you can get by by being 'mostly gluten-free'. It's like being pregnant. You either are or not - there's no 'kind of' or 'most the time'. It's also important to know that gluten sensitivity and being Coeliac is completely different, too. You can be sensitive to gluten  yet still have a negative Coeliac test result. There's more information on gluten and thyroid disease in Chapter 4.

## Other Food

Other food sensitivities with Hashimoto's are also common - dairy, nuts, eggs, nightshades, citrus foods etc. You can try an elimination diet whereby you remove them for a period of time and then reintroduce them one by one and keep a close eye on your symptoms to see which are your issue. Keep a food diary for a few weeks and note any symptoms or complaints and see if they correlate to any foods eaten. More information on this is given in Chapter 7. Common dietary changes with Hashimoto's patients include gluten-free, dairy free, AIP, Keto and more. I'll be delving in to the most popular one, gluten-free here, but for others you'll find a wealth of information online and in thyroid specific cookbooks.

## Adrenal Fatigue

It is also important to check your adrenal health. I've covered adrenal fatigue (hypothalamic-pituitary axis dysfunction) in more detail further on in this book, but for now I'll just say that I believe most hypothyroid patients have some degree of adrenal dysfunction and although it's not a condition widely recognised by conventional medicine just yet, I do feel it will be in the future. The adrenal glands manage our response to stress and danger and with Hashimoto's, we often have inflammation or other disruptions going on in the body that the adrenals react to with the stress response. Over time, this can be just as debilitating as hypothyroidism in its own right. I've covered it a lot more in Chapter 4 so won't repeat it here.

## Gut Health

Having a leaky gut, yeast overgrowth (Candida), GERD, acid reflux or other digestive/abdominal issues or complaints is also very common with Hashimoto's, as the gut lining becomes compromised over time, or yeast becomes overgrown, opening us up to issues such as food sensitivities, reflux, constipation and even difficulty absorbing nutrients and vitamins. Low levels of iron, B12 and Vitamin D can be a sign and must be addressed. Each one can cause their own set of symptoms on top of your hypothyroid symptoms. The best way to treat leaky gut I've found, is by seeking out a functional doctor to tailor a treatment programme to your needs. You'll find more information in Chapter 4 about this.

## Blood Sugar

Hashimoto's also puts us at an increased risk of blood sugar imbalances or glycaemic impairments[6]. Before I realised the importance of managing my blood sugar levels, I would get 'hangry' (hungry and angry) several times a day, as my blood sugar would drop after a big spike from the sugar and carbs I was eating a lot of. Other signs of blood sugar imbalances include headaches, feeling faint and dizzy, feeling hungry again quickly after eating, feeling tired, grouchy and irritable. Until a couple of years ago, I wasn't aware that these low blood sugar moments were putting a lot of stress on my adrenals and could also be contributing to my high thyroid antibodies. Hello worse symptoms!

Since realising that I needed to adjust my diet to allow more protein and less sugar and carbs, my low blood sugar bouts, irritable moods, groggy feeling and slumps are gone. If I do slip up, I feel sick, irritable, get a headache and generally just *urgh*. It's really not good. Ideas for well-balanced and thyroid healthy meals can be found in *The 30-Minute Thyroid Cookbook* by Emily Kyle.

Blood sugar imbalances place even more stress on our adrenal glands, which isn't good at all, seeing as so many of us with hypothyroidism have 'adrenal fatigue' as it is, because of the stress it puts on our body (and also often our mind). When your blood sugar levels drop below normal, your adrenal glands respond by secreting cortisol. This cortisol then tells the liver to produce more glucose, which brings blood sugar levels back to normal. Doing this repeatedly can cause abnormal cortisol output and can suppress pituitary function.

The glycaemic index is a measurement of how quickly we burn food, and carbohydrates have a very quick burn rate. Because of this, when eaten, they cause a spike in our blood sugar. Despite there being a general myth that carbohydrates keep us fuller for longer, after eating them, we actually often tend to become hungry again in less than an hour! I was always confused as to why I could be starving within an hour after eating a whole bowl of pasta or a jacket potato. It makes sense now. World-renowned Dr Datis Kharrazian explains in his book *Why Do I STILL Have Thyroid Symptoms? When My Lab Tests Are Normal* that if you feel sleepy or want sugar or sweets after a meal, it's a sign you've ate too much carbs and a sign of low blood sugar or insulin resistance – blood sugar imbalances.

This is why more protein-rich diets are often better for us. Fat and protein have a slower burn rate. The energy from protein is released more slowly and gradually and so doesn't raise blood sugar levels as quickly as carbs. They also keep us fuller for longer.

## How I Got My Own Hashimoto's in to Remission

I brought my own levels of thyroid antibodies down from more than 1300 to almost nothing i.e. back within the normal range. From June 2015 to February 2019 they dropped consistently. Within the first three years my TPOAB level went from more than 1300 to just 244. Everything I implemented in that time included: changing from Levothyroxine to NDT medication, supplementing Vitamin D, Vitamin C, Selenium, iron, going gluten-free, stopping the yo-yo dieting and cutting of calories which was putting more stress on my body and making me more sick and instead focusing on nutrition and wholesome foods, and stopping the exercise that was also contributing to adrenal stress. I went from intense cardio to gentle walking.

From April 2018 to November 2018, they dropped even further from 174 to 144, during which time I started supplementing Magnesium Citrate, probiotics, Zinc, B Vitamins, digestive enzymes, drinking bone broths, addressing my leaky gut and candida, which in turn addressed the oestrogen dominance and adrenal dysfunction.

And from November 2018 to February 2019, they dropped even further and I also tested TGAB (the other type of thyroid antibody test) for the first time too, which was also low. Both were now within normal range and all I had done in those last few months was started a L-Tyrosine supplement on guidance from my functional medicine practitioner, cleaned up my diet even more so and increased my exercise frequency so that I was taking long walks in nature daily. I also started dance classes a few times a week.

It's important that I say here just how individual we all are and how we all have our own 'thyroid jigsaw puzzles' to piece back together. Whilst my pieces consisted of specific supplementation, dietary changes and more, yours will most likely be made up on your own combination of puzzle pieces. It's your responsibility to advocate for yourself in locating which things make up your thyroid jigsaw. What worked for me may or may not work for you. Having a functional medicine practitioner guide me on the interventions and changes I needed to make, made a big difference and she managed what dosage of supplements I took. Again, what each of us need or don't need can vary a lot.

## Let's Recap on Hashimoto's

So addressing Hashimoto's by considering your gut health, infections, adrenals, vitamin levels, blood sugar imbalances and food sensitivities (mainly gluten) can help to calm down the attack and lessen symptoms. Some even claim to set their Hashimoto's into remission and no longer need thyroid medication, though I don't believe this to be that common. So many of us find out we have it at such a late stage, that our thyroid is already severely damaged and thyroid hormone output affected. If you are interested in setting your Hashimoto's into remission though, take a look at Thyroid Pharmacist Izabella Wentz for more information. She has dedicated her career to sharing what helped her do just this.

## What Else Causes Hypothyroidism?

Besides Hashimoto's, there are other causes for hypothyroidism.

### Genetics

The thyroid gland may not develop properly at birth, known as congenital hypothyroidism. This is a condition resulting from an absent or underdeveloped thyroid gland, or one that has developed but cannot make enough thyroid hormone. The term 'congenital' means that the condition is present at birth. For some babies, their thyroid gland does not form in its normal position in the neck. In others, the gland does not develop at all. And for others, it is simply just underdeveloped. The British Thyroid Foundation estimate that 1 child in every 3,500-4,000 is born with hypothyroidism in the UK.[7]

The thyroid gland may also fail later in life, which is more common. Dr Barry Durrant-Peatfield describes this as it being 'programmed to fail', in his book *Your Thyroid and how to keep it healthy.. The Great Thyroid Scandal and How to Survive it*. This basically means that it is essentially a ticking time-bomb as to when it will fail, but that it was always going to. You may notice a pattern in your family such as signs of the condition starting in the twenties or at middle-aged, for example.

It appears that having Down Syndrome[8] increases the risk of having accompanying hypothyroidism.

## Radioactive Iodine Therapy and Radiation

A treatment often used for hyperthyroidism (an overactive thyroid), RAI results in hypothyroidism, where the thyroid is permanently disabled from working at all or working less than it used to.

Radiation therapy to the neck area, such as when treating certain cancers, can also lead to hypothyroidism. Radiation can damage thyroid cells, which can make it more difficult for the thyroid to produce thyroid hormones.

## Surgery

Surgery to remove the thyroid gland will obviously lead to hypothyroidism. If only part of the thyroid is removed, the remaining *may* still be able to produce enough thyroid hormone alone, but commonly doesn't, so medication for life is needed to replace the hormones that are missing.

## The Environment

Toxins are all around us. Chlorine and Fluorine are big ones for thyroid disease, as well as Mercury. Many people have mercury in their dental fillings, which have been said to contribute to hypothyroidism, due to the way it can affect selenium levels, with selenium being very vital to thyroid function. If you think your dental amalgams may be contributing to your thyroid problems, then you should definitely discuss this with your dentist.

A scalloped tongue can be a sign of excess toxins in the body and my own enlarged, scalloped tongue has gone down in size since improving detoxification in my own body.

Dr Barry Durrant-Peatfield also explains in his book *Your Thyroid and how to keep it healthy.. The Great Thyroid Scandal and How to Survive it,* how high dosage cortisones, given for asthma and rheumatoid arthritis for example, such as dioxins and PCBs, can remain in the body for a long time. Years even. And apparently they can affect the liver, reproductive processes, immune system, adrenals and thyroid function. Other medications such as those for heart conditions, cancer, psychiatric conditions, lithium etc. can also affect thyroid function.

Goitrogenic and soy foods also suppress thyroid function, though likely wouldn't cause hypothyroidism on their own unless eaten excessively. The general consensus for goitrogenic foods such as brussel sprouts, cabbage, broccoli, cauliflower, kale, spinach, sweet potatoes etc. is to ensure they're fully cooked before eating, to reduce the goitrogenic properties.

## Deficiencies

Deficiencies in certain vitamins, minerals and nutrients can also lead to hypothyroidism. Iodine is a well-recognised one, as adequate iodine is needed for proper thyroid function. Supplementing iodine is controversial, as many sources say to only supplement if you definitely need it.

Adequate selenium levels are another important part of adequate thyroid function. It promotes energy and the conversion of T4 to T3, so low levels of it can cause low levels thyroid hormone.

## Contraceptive Pill

Many functional medicine practitioners such as Dr Datis Kharrazian and Dr Jolene Brighten, state that too much oestrogen, often caused by the contraceptive pill, can cause hypothyroidism.

Contraceptive pills can also deplete vitamins and nutrients, leading to deficiencies that increase thyroid hormones binding meaning that less is available for use by cells.

Excess oestrogen can also affect how much thyroid hormone is used by the body. I struggled a lot with heavy, painful and disruptive periods from a young age. Doctors proceeded to put me on the contraceptive pill to help this, which it did to a certain extent, but being on the pill and having an undiagnosed thyroid problem led to monthly, debilitating hormonal migraines. When I came off the pill, the migraines improved quite a bit. The contraceptive pill was only masking my hormonal balance instead of addressing it.

## Adrenal Dysfunction

A failing thyroid gland can cause the adrenals to become stressed and fatigued. But what if you had adrenal dysfunction first, that *caused or encouraged* hypothyroidism? What if the adrenal system is damaged in such a way as to interfere with thyroid function and hormone uptake?

## Trauma

Direct damage such as whiplash, being roughly handled around the throat, hitting your chin on the dashboard in a car accident etc. can understandably lead to a damaged thyroid gland and thus, affected output of hormone.

## Central Hypothyroidism

Although rare, if something is wrong with the pituitary gland, this can interfere with the production of thyroid hormones. The pituitary gland produces TSH, which tells the thyroid how much hormones it should make and release. If something is wrong with the pituitary gland, then thyroid hormone production and release will be affected, causing hypothyroidism.

A similar problem can be of the hypothalamus too. Although rare as well, hypothyroidism can occur if the hypothalamus, situated in the brain, does not produce enough TRH, which tells the pituitary to release TSH.

## The Tests You Need to Be Having Done

As well as being tested for Hashimoto's, you should have other tests conducted upon diagnosis to give a comprehensive view of things. Hopefully your doctor has made the diagnosis based on a full thyroid panel, though I know many still do not. I always suggest retrieving a printed copy of all test results you ever receive and keeping them in a neat folder at home so that you can refer back to them whenever you need. There are also many apps now available so you can manage your thyroid health via your smartphone.

Your doctor should always be testing as many of these as possible: TSH, Free T3, Free T4, TPOAB, TGAB and Reverse T3 (though Reverse T3 is often hard to obtain as many labs just don't test it). They form the thyroid panel, and, despite what many doctors will claim, TSH alone is definitely not accurate enough to go by for your diagnosis, treatment and management of hypothyroidism. TSH is a pituitary hormone, not a thyroid hormone. It serves as an average read out over the previous four to six weeks of your thyroid levels.

**Let's look at TSH like this:**

TSH (Thyroid Stimulating Hormone) is a pituitary hormone that sends a signal to the thyroid gland. It is produced by the pituitary gland.

### Hypothalamus (sends signal to) → Pituitary (sends signal to) → Thyroid

With a healthy thyroid, the pituitary gland knocks on the thyroid's door, signalling it to work and produce so much of certain hormones. It does this by releasing TSH. The thyroid answers the door and does what it's told by the pituitary by releasing the correct amount of thyroid hormone. Therefore, the pituitary gland isn't having to knock too much, which equals a low TSH. This is good. In a person with hypothyroidism, the pituitary gland knocks on the door of the thyroid gland, trying to give orders, but the thyroid ignores it. It doesn't respond. The pituitary gland therefore bangs harder on the door, as the thyroid continues to ignore it, and doesn't produce the hormones it should be. This equals a high TSH. This isn't good.

Theoretically, if you put the hormones your body is lacking and thyroid is failing to produce, in to your body, the TSH will come down, as the pituitary doesn't need to knock on the door so much, as it can see that the body is getting the hormones it needs. Doctors see the TSH being low as your body having what it needs.

Another analogy you could use when your doctor tells you your TSH is fine, but you don't feel 'fine' is this: *Would you be happy with a heating engineer telling you your central heating is working fine, just because the thermostat reading is normal, when the radiators are cold and the house is freezing?*

Having a 'fine' TSH is one thing, however, your body actually performing properly is another. As already established, TSH is s a pituitary hormone, not a thyroid hormone. It does not tell you your actual thyroid hormone levels. You need Free T3 and Free T4 testing to check these.

Therefore, you can still feel rubbish with a 'normal' TSH because:

- Your body could be failing to convert the T4 (thyroxine, also known as Levothyroxine and Synthroid) to T3, which makes you feel rubbish, still. T4 is the storage hormone, T3 is the active hormone, what is actually *used*. TSH doesn't tell you if you're converting adequately.
- Your Free T3 and T4 levels could be below optimal or at the bottom of the range.
- Your TSH may be 'in range' but not 'optimal'.

- As proposed by Stop The Thyroid Madness, your adrenal glands could be dysfunctioning or you have low iron levels, leading to T3 not getting to all your cells, organs and muscles etc. adequately[9]. They report that this can show as a low TSH, but high Free T3 levels on blood results. This is referred to as 'pooling' by Stop The Thyroid Madness but isn't a widely recognised theory elsewhere.

The next time your TSH is 'fine' and you still feel unwell, one of these could well be why. Many thyroid patients find that whilst their TSH is OK, their Free T3 and Free T4, or even Reverse T3 isn't optimal and so they still feel unwell. Now you know all of this, please don't stay undiagnosed, under-medicated or be dismissed due to just having TSH tested. Get a copy of your test results, look for yourself and begin to understand what they mean.

## Optimal Levels

So, you managed to find out what your test results say? Great! Now we can look at where they *should* be, to be considered optimal.

It's a term I, and so many other sources for thyroid information, use a lot. What *are* optimal thyroid levels? A lot of conventional medicine doctors and endocrinologists refuse to acknowledge that it's not just about falling 'in range', but it's *where* in range you fall that matters. It matters entirely.

Put simply, when your doctor runs a test and you get the results, optimal levels are the results that most thyroid patients state they feel best at. This is a more specific place within a given range. So, it's not just about falling in range that matters. It's *where* you fall in range that can affect how you feel.

You'll find that many thyroid advocacies, functional medicine practitioners and research agree that a TSH of 0.5-2 is considered optimal. In 2002, the National Academy of Clinical Biochemistry (NACB) issued new guidelines for the diagnosis and monitoring of thyroid disease, which reported that the TSH reference range was too wide and actually included people with thyroid disease, thus making it inaccurate. When more sensitive screening was done, which excluded people with thyroid disease, 95% of the population tested had a TSH level between 0.4 and 2.5. As a result, the NACB recommended reducing the reference range to those levels[10]. Furthermore, the third National Health and Nutrition Examination Survey (NHANES III) screened 17,353 subjects from 1988 to 1994 and excluded those with diseases or factors known to affect thyroid function too. In the resultant 'normal' population of 13,344 subjects, 95% had TSH levels that fell between 0.3 and 2.5, which is almost identical to the findings of the NACB above, again, backing up a TSH below 2.5. [11] NHS England guidelines from November 2018 also clearly state that TSH should be between 0.4-1.5 when treated with Levothyroxine medications.[12]

This optimal range for TSH means that a lot of thyroid patients feel their best when their TSH is between 0.5 and 2, but we now know that TSH alone isn't accurate, so what about those other levels? Well, Free T3 in the top quarter of the given range is often recommended[13], with a Free T4 mid-range or a little higher. I can vouch for this information and confirm that I do indeed feel best when my levels are all within these optimal subsections of ranges. Occasionally, my Free T4 may drop slightly but as long as my Free T3 is high within the range, I feel well. Please note, that as these optimal levels fall within the range your doctor is already using, they cannot equal *hyper*thyroidism or overmedication.

It is important to understand that different labs and doctors use different ranges, so you must interpret your results *individually*; don't compare them to anyone else's. A Free T4 at 14, with a range of 9-19, is mid-range for example, but a Free T4 at 11 is mid-range for a range of 7.5-14.5. So, both are considered optimal readings, even though they're different numbers. You must look at your result in comparison to the given range, usually stated in brackets, beside it. Where does it fall?

It's important to be aware that a suppressed TSH alone doesn't necessarily mean you're hyperthyroid or over medicated. If your Free T3 and Free T4 are still within range then they show that your thyroid hormone levels aren't too high. Explaining to your doctor that you wish to see how you feel with thyroid hormone levels higher up in range should be a reasonable enough request, but it's just making sure you have those Free T3 and Free T4 levels tested and not just TSH, which is often the tricky part.

## What You Need To Know About Doing Thyroid Blood Tests

In regards to T4-only medication such as Levothyroxine and Synthroid, they only have a half-life of around five to nine days, which means that once you've become stable on a dose, it takes around a week for half of that dose to clear the body and blood levels to reflect this. This is why, when some people decide to stop taking their thyroid medication, they feel fine for the first week or so. (Please note - I don't recommend stopping your medication without a plan to replace those thyroid hormones at all).

Therefore, whether you take T4-only medication *right* before your blood test or blood sample is taken, or haven't taken it for up to two days beforehand, your TSH levels and Free T3 levels *should* still be the same, but free T4 may well show a peak two hours after taking T4 medications.

According to Thyroid Manager[14]:

*"Serum T4 (Free T4) concentrations peak two to four hours after an oral dose and remain above normal for approximately six hours in patients receiving daily replacement therapy."*

*For this reason, thyroid expert Richard Shames, MD has the following recommendation:*

*"I absolutely recommend that patients have any morning blood tests evaluating the thyroid before taking any thyroid medication."*

So, if you were to take your T4-only thyroid medication before a thyroid blood draw, your Free T4 levels could come out elevated, leading to your doctor lowering the medication dosage, when you don't actually need it lowering. So to get a reading of your Free T4 level that is reflective of most the day, you should hold fire on taking your medication until after the blood test.

Now, if you're taking a thyroid medication that contains T3, such as NDT or T3 synthetic Liothyronine, it's important to be aware that T3 has a half-life of around eighteen hours. Straight after taking a T3 containing medication, the TSH level begins to fall and then stays suppressed for as long as five hours. Free T3 levels also increase after taking T3 medication and hit a peak after three to four hours. This means that if you were to take your T3 containing thyroid medication within five hours prior to getting your thyroid tests done, your test results may imply that you are overmedicated when you're not, or even that your levels are within range or optimal, when you're actually under-medicated. So, it can affect your ability to get an accurate result and adjust your dosage accurately.

Therefore, you're best to hold off taking this medication until after the blood draw. I take my thyroid medication with me so that I can take it straight after the blood test, otherwise I can start to feel unwell.

You may also wonder if you need to fast before a blood test.

In terms of fasting, most doctors tell thyroid patients that it's not necessary to fast before a blood test. However, researchers have found[15] that after eating, our TSH level becomes suppressed. This means that a high TSH could instead look much lower after eating, and borderline levels no longer borderline. As so many doctors use the TSH level to decide if a patient is adequately treated, or in need of more or less thyroid medication, this could result in patients having their thyroid medication wrongly altered, or even being told that their 'borderline' hypothyroidism is now 'normal', resulting in some thyroid patients being inadequately treated for their thyroid condition. All because they ate before their test.

Therefore, your TSH level is likely to be at its highest and most reflective of its underlying status, when tested *after* fasting, *in the early morning.* Another thing to keep in mind is the *time* at which your blood is drawn for thyroid testing.

Each time you have your thyroid tests done, you should aim for it to always be done at the same time, and under the same circumstances (i.e. fasting), so they're as accurate and comparable as possible. Given that you shouldn't take your medication until after the test, as early as possible in the morning and before 9am is preferable. This is because thyroid hormone levels have a circadian rhythm with a peak at night, so Dr Geracioti suggests[16] that blood tests for hypothyroidism be done before 9am in order to not miss subclinical hypothyroidism and have as accurate results as possible.

If you're also one of the thyroid patients who take the supplement biotin, it is also worth knowing that this can cause falsely elevated thyroid levels on test results, making you look overmedicated or hyperthyroid when you're not. Therefore, it is advised to not take biotin supplements for at least 48-hours before a thyroid blood test. Though some people prefer to go up to two weeks to make sure it doesn't influence results.

Many people worry if being unwell at the time of a thyroid blood draw affects the test results. Being unwell *could* affect test results temporarily, as sometimes, infections or a bout of an inflammatory condition can alter results until the illness resolves. So, if you receive an unexpected result when unwell, it is probably wise to retest after you've recovered to rule it out as a cause. Also, as diarrhoea can interfere with the absorption of your thyroid medication, this could affect your thyroid hormone levels and any testing, so this form of sickness could affect results. Being on your period whilst testing thyroid hormone levels isn't known to cause any issues or affect results, but if you're feeling particularly unwell from your period then you may wish to have blood drawn when you feel better. Especially if you already lose a lot of blood with menstruation, as heavy periods can go hand in hand with hypothyroidism.

## How Often To Test?

In terms of how often you should be having your thyroid tests conducted, once every six to twelve months is standard if your levels are optimal and you feel well (once in winter and once in summer can be a good idea, as external temperatures can alter our need for thyroid hormone). Every two months is more common if you're still adjusting dosage and having symptoms. Some patients need their dosage altering as the weather gets colder, and again when it warms up, to reflect an increase or decrease in demand for thyroid hormone, due to external temperatures.

When first starting thyroid medication for hypothyroidism, most doctors recommend testing thyroid levels again about four to six weeks after the start of the treatment, to determine if the dose of medication is correct, but waiting eight weeks can allow the medication to finish building in the body and supply a more accurate reading. When your thyroid gland isn't working properly, thus leading to hypothyroidism, it's incredibly important to correct the low levels of thyroid hormone with frequent and thorough testing.

## Chapter Recap:

- The spoon theory can be a good way to understand altered energy levels and how to look at managing them.

- Hashimoto's is behind most cases of hypothyroidism and treating it often involves more than just medication alone.

- There are other causes of hypothyroidism besides Hashimoto's.

- TSH alone isn't accurate and a full thyroid panel really ought to be tested every time to ensure the most comprehensive view of your thyroid health is obtained.

- Optimal levels are often the biggest piece to a thyroid patient's jigsaw puzzle. Optimising treatment can solve many symptoms and issues. The studies and research to back these up are shown at the end of the book.

- Knowing how to prepare for blood tests can help you ensure your results are as accurate as possible so treatment is optimised.

# Chapter 3: Thyroid Medication Options

*"Taking thyroid medication does not make you weak."* -
*Rachel Hill, The Invisible Hypothyroidism*

Although many doctors will not tell you (and often do not know themselves), there *are* more options for treating your thyroid condition than just T4-only medication such as Levothyroxine or Synthroid. In fact, a lot of conventional doctors don't even seem to be aware that they can treat hypothyroidism with more than synthetic T4-only drugs.

So, if you're one of the many thyroid patients who are on a T4-only medication such as Levothyroxine or Synthroid, and don't feel much better, I'm about to tell you how a different medication may well do a better job.

## How Do Thyroid Medications Differ?

Let's start with a bit of science.

A healthy thyroid gland would be giving you five hormones you need and these are: T1, T2, T3, T4 and Calcitonin. T1 is thought to play a role in keeping your thyroid function in check and also is believed to influence the heart. T2 may play a role in converting T4 to T3. It also likely has an impact on metabolism and burning fat and is effective in increasing liver metabolism and that of the heart. Referred to as the 'active hormone', T3 has the greatest effect on the body's energy levels and overall health and well-being and is required in optimal amounts for good mental health, ability to cope with stress and emotional stability. T4 is referred to as the 'storage hormone' and its main function is to convert to T3, mainly in the liver, to both active T3 and Reverse T3. T4 is involved in brain function also. Calcitonin is secreted from the thyroid when blood levels are high in Calcium. It acts to lower levels of Calcium in the blood and stops the release of more Calcium from your bones into the blood. Because of this, it's said to be effective in the prevention of osteoporosis.

So, you can see why it may be beneficial to take a thyroid medication that replaces all or at least the two most important (T3 and T4) of these thyroid hormones, when our thyroid glands go caput and we develop hypothyroidism. Well, a lot of conventional medicine practitioners would not agree and favour T4-only medicines.

## T4-only

Most conventional doctors believe that we only need to replace the T4, as we only require tiny amounts of T1, T2 and Calcitonin anyway, and our body will convert some of the T4 to T3, to replace that thyroid hormone too. And this seems simple enough, right? *Wrong.* While some people do well on T4-only medications, many patients fail to convert the T4 into T3, so when they take T4-only medication, they still feel rubbish. And this is something many doctors are refusing to acknowledge.

A conversion issue can be caused by an enzyme called iodothyronine deiodinase that is either deficient or not compatible for some people and is important in the activation and deactivation of thyroid hormones. T4 is converted into T3 by deiodinase activity. A problem with this can therefore cause conversion issues, where TSH can look 'fine', as well as Free T4, but with a low Free T3 and continued hypothyroid symptoms and development of other health conditions (such as mental health and heart/blood pressure problems).

Another cause could be adrenal dysfunction, or vitamin deficiencies such as iron or selenium, and so by addressing these, you may fix the conversion problem, but many other people simply have a problem converting and don't know why. So obviously, they will benefit from taking a thyroid medication that gives them direct T3, instead of relying on their body to convert the T4.

## T3-only

Instead of being on T4-only, you could be on T3-only medication which skips that conversion stage too. But as you have no T4 (the storage hormone) to convert to T3 throughout the day for you, you may have to dose it more often, such as three or even four times a day. Still, some thyroid patients do feel an improvement over being on T4-only medication alone.

## T3 and T4 Combination Therapy

There is also the option of taking both T4 and T3 together, to try and mimic more closely what the thyroid gland would be producing, if it was working properly. Thyroid patients who have tried this do often report much better results than using T4-only on its own, as it gives you that direct T3 and doesn't rely on your body to convert it. Both of these are synthetic hormones though (made by chemical synthesis to imitate a natural product) so for some, don't quite work as well as 'natural thyroid' options, which are up next.

## Compounded Thyroid Medication

Compounded thyroid medication offers the advantage of being made without any fillers, which can be useful if you do not tolerate them well, such as gluten or lactose. The amounts of T3 and T4 are usually similar to NDT (mentioned below), but doctors can order for the amount of each to be adjusted to make the exact dosage your own body needs. It is essentially more personalised than regular NDT. This can be the answer for those who do not feel well on synthetic T3, T4 or standard NDT medications.

Most compounded thyroid medications are 'immediate release' versions, which means that they release the active medication immediately after taking, but compounding pharmacists are also able to make sustained release versions, where the medication is released more gradually; continuously throughout the day.

## NDT (Natural Desiccated Thyroid)

Natural Desiccated Thyroid is most often dried porcine thyroid gland and gives you the five hormones your own thyroid would be giving you if it was perfectly healthy; T1, T2, T3, T4 and Calcitonin. A lot of patients who've tried T4-only medicine, T4 and T3 together, or even just T3 on its own, say they have even better results with NDT because of how much closer its composition is to that of a healthy gland's output. However, as with everything, we're all different.

Most people seem to dose NDT twice a day, taking half their dose in the morning and the other half mid-afternoon to mimic what their own thyroid would be doing more closely. However, I haven't noticed a difference whether I take mine once daily or twice daily. NDT removes the need to rely on the body converting thyroid hormones.

Obviously, NDT is a tricky decision for thyroid patients who are vegetarian or otherwise do not eat meat or pork, but it's all down to your personal situation. Over the counter bovine NDT can be found for those who cannot eat pork.

## Changing Thyroid Medication

Now, you may have read all of that and thought *"Brilliant. How do I change to this NDT or T3 medication?"* Well, the hardest part is trying to convince your doctor to prescribe anything other than T4-only medication. The vast majority of conventional doctors have been trained to stick to T4 synthetics (there's a whole, complicated history behind thyroid medications[17]), therefore many patients these days are unfortunately having to go private or even self-source NDT or T3 (such as buying it online), just to get the medication they need to function like a normal human being again. It's all very controversial and a bit of a mess! After seeing numerous NHS GPs here in England and having NDT refused again and again, I eventually turned to self-sourcing my NDT and let me tell you – it was no easy decision.

Of course, it is risky. Of course, buying any medication online wasn't ideal. It is *far* from ideal. It didn't exactly make me feel great about myself. And of course, you must be so clued up and well-read in how to use such medication if your doctor has no idea how to dose it themselves, but I can't deny that it changed my life - heck, even *saved* my life - and the effects NDT has had on me has even changed my own GPs idea on the medication. When I began self-sourcing, he happily supported me using it and monitored me with regular full thyroid panel blood tests but he wouldn't prescribe it still. So eventually, after a few years, I went private and obtained a private prescription for NDT medication from a private doctor. Thus, ending my need to self-source. However, not everyone can afford to go private, so I count myself as rather lucky in this regard.

Thyroid advocates and charities here in the UK especially are still campaigning for more routine prescribing of NDT and T3 medications on the NHS. There's a long journey ahead! Just please do not take self-sourcing lightly. It comes with a lot of risks and I would be deceiving if I didn't stress that. It is always best to get any medication prescribed and managed by a medical professional. Just be aware that you're more likely to get T3 and NDT medication from a private doctor or functional medicine doctor, more specifically. It's becoming harder as time goes on, to get these options on the NHS. If you're struggling to find a doctor who will consider prescribing alternatives to just T4-only medication, you could also try asking your pharmacist if they know of any doctors who prescribe them.

Now, after all this talk about NDT, don't get me wrong regarding the other thyroid medication options. I am not suggesting that NDT or T3 synthetics are the only way forward, and some thyroid patients *do* do well on T4-only medication, but the problem is that doctors need to be treating patients based on their own individual needs, symptoms and reactions to medication. The best thyroid medicine is the one that works best for *that* particular person. This should include T3 and NDT medications, as well as T4-only.

## How Long Will It Take Me to Feel Well Again?

As well as feeling relieved that they finally have an answer for why they've been feeling so unwell, patients often say that they also feel impatient about waiting for their thyroid medication to 'kick in' too. So, how long after starting thyroid hormone replacement medication, will it take for you to get back to how well you used to feel?

In short, I can't tell you. I wish I could though. I really do. But sadly, I am not psychic (though how cool would that be if I was?)

The thing is, it's different for each person. Why? Because the point at which we finally get that diagnosis and the medication that our body so desperately needs, is commonly so late in the progression of the condition, that we also then have other issues that now need addressing too.

You see, whilst some people start their thyroid medication and within a few weeks feel great, many of us don't feel loads better this quickly. But please don't fret, because you can feel well again. It just takes time to address what's going on inside your body.

Each person's thyroid journey is very unique. Some people find that their first try of thyroid medication alone does very well in bringing them back to good health, but for others, they find that they either require medication dosage adjustments (i.e. the initial dose of medication given isn't enough), a switch to a different type of medication and/or some further help or problem solving in other areas.

For a lot of us with hypothyroidism and especially autoimmune hypothyroidism, we also have issues such as adrenal problems, vitamin deficiencies (or low levels still causing issues and symptoms), gut issues, sex hormone imbalances and even food sensitivities. And these will need addressing too, as covered in Chapter 2.

It is possible to live a good quality, full life with hypothyroidism however, but each person needs to piece together their own thyroid jigsaw puzzle to figure out what needs addressing in their case.

Myself for example, I've had to address a change in medication from Levothyroxine to Natural Desiccated Thyroid, low ferritin, low Vitamin D, high Hashimoto's antibodies, 'adrenal fatigue', sex hormone imbalances (oestrogen dominance), gluten sensitivity, leaky gut, candida and more. But by addressing each of these issues, I've gotten closer and closer to the level of health that I remember having prior to developing autoimmune hypothyroidism. It really is like a jigsaw puzzle and each person's will be made up of different pieces for them to address and slot back in to place.

So, how long will it take you to feel well again? It's going to depend on how many aspects you need to address, how well you take control of your health and advocate for yourself and how your individual body reacts and adjusts. Do bear in mind that, often, the longer you've been unwell without diagnosis and medication, the more likely you'll have multiple issues to address, as untreated hypothyroidism/Hashimoto's can send other things out of whack over time.

## Are You Taking Your Thyroid Medication Properly?

Advice on how to take your thyroid medication, whether given by doctors, pharmacists or even on medication box leaflets, can be confusing and contradictory. But it's important to know how to take it correctly to get the most out of it.

Most of us read the leaflet that comes with a new medication, paying particular attention to the listed side effects and interactions section, but it's important to be aware of how other things you eat, drink or medications you take, can affect the absorption and effectiveness of your thyroid medications. You should always take your thyroid medications at least one hour away from any other food or drink (excluding water), medications (especially antacids, antidepressants and antibiotics) and supplements, leaving four hours between thyroid medication and supplements containing calcium, oestrogen, magnesium and iron. Not doing so can affect how much of the thyroid hormone in your medication you absorb, meaning you're not getting as much as you should be. And this can affect how you feel on them.

You should also aim to take your thyroid medication at the same time every day, and if you take T3 containing thyroid medication, this is often multi-dosed throughout the day, as mentioned previously in the section on T3 medications. If you're on T4-only medicine then you may benefit from taking this at night but this isn't recommended with T3 containing preparations as it could keep you up at night.

It is also worth noting that coffee has been reported to affect the absorption of T4-only thyroid medication[18], which is why thyroid patients should wait at least an hour after taking their medication before drinking any coffee, too. To get around this, an option could be to take medication at night, though remember this is only recommended for T4. Some studies have shown[19] that taking Levothyroxine at bedtime may improve absorption. It also allows for you to have your morning cup of coffee without worrying about it affecting your thyroid medication.

Your medications can also become less effective if they're past their expiry date, so always check this when you're first given them and make a mental note (or physical note) about when it'll need replacing. Ensure you never run out and never miss or skip doses as this can cause you to feel unwell as hypothyroid symptoms creep back in. Stopping thyroid medication altogether can even be life threatening. If you've been prescribed a specific brand or type of thyroid medication which is working for you and you get on well with, make sure that you're always given the same one, as some thyroid patients are given a generic substitute in place of their usual and end up feeling unwell again.

You may find that doctors and patients alike have many views on whether you should multi-dose thyroid medication, take them on an empty stomach, with other medication or even at night, but in my opinion, it's just safest to use common sense and let your body absorb as much of it as possible before eating, drinking or taking other things. *It just makes sense.* And following these practises won't do any harm to you but can only benefit you.

# Tips For Remembering To Take Your Meds

## Use Your Phone

Setting an alarm on your phone, putting reminders in your phone calendar or keeping a list of medications and times to take them can be effective.

## Use Every day Routines

What definitely helps me, is tying the need to take any medication or supplement with an activity I do each day. At bedtime I take certain supplements, just before I shower I take my thyroid medication and with dinner I take my Vitamin D.

## Leave Notes

You could leave yourself notes on the mirror, fridge, or even on top of your phone if it's the first thing you check every morning!

## Use Pill Boxes

Pill boxes are probably the most traditional way to remember tablets.

## Ask Friends and Family to Remind You

Some of your friends and family may also take medications, so you could create a group that helps to remind each other.

If you live with someone, make them aware of your meds schedule and ask them to try and remind you too.

## Keep it Visible

"Out of sight, out of mind," is a phrase we've all heard before and it's even true when it comes to remembering to take your meds! Keep them somewhere you spend a lot of time or go to everyday.

## Levothyroxine - 'The Gold Standard' - My Experience

I was prescribed T4-only Levothyroxine when first diagnosed, just like most thyroid patients and I was honestly really hopeful about it working. In fact, after a few weeks, I did start to see a difference as my energy levels rose and I began feeling happier and more positive. But it was short lived. After just two weeks of this amazing feeling, I crashed to even lower than before I'd started Levothyroxine. My symptoms came back with a vengeance, new symptoms were multiplying quickly and I soon became concerned. I went back and forth to the doctor's surgery, where they proclaimed my thyroid levels (just TSH and Free T4 at this time) to be 'perfectly normal' repeatedly. Yet they had no answer for why I was feeling so rubbish.

At one point I went back to ask them to retest as I had read online and in some books that taking my thyroid medication before a test could cause a false 'high', indicating I was doing better than I was, so I wanted to retest levels with me taking the medication *after* the test. The doctor reluctantly agreed, but alas, the results came back about the same. I just knew that something wasn't right and I just knew that it was my thyroid condition. After all, you know your own body better than anyone else.

After reading further into hypothyroidism and discovering various resources such as Mary Shomon, Hypothyroid Mom and Stop The Thyroid Madness (which was the kick up the backside I needed to advocate for myself), I decided that I wanted to try NDT, feeling as if I was one of the many thyroid patients not converting my T4 medication into T3, so I went back to the doctor again to ask to be prescribed it, knowing that my chances were slim.

Well, it could *not* have gone any worse. The GP became more and more angry as I went through each of my bullet points on a quivering post-it note I had scrunched up in my hand. I rattled off various points:

*"I would like a full thyroid panel testing. I would like to come off the contraceptive pill because I feel it's masking my hormonal issues. I would like printouts of my test results from the past year and most importantly, I want to try natural desiccated thyroid."*

My oh my was he angry. He batted every single request down without any room for discussion. Not letting me speak, he said that testing TSH and Free T4 was 'enough', that I was 'optimally treated' on Levothyroxine so all my symptoms must be in my head, that I was 'prime age' to fall pregnant so must remain on my contraceptive pill and definitely could not have NDT, since it's very outdated and I 'shouldn't believe what I read on the world wide web'.

I corrected him to say I'd read multiple studies and books and referenced to them but he became even more flustered, produced a prescription for another type of contraceptive pill and pushed me out the door. He was probably quite pleased in how he handled it.

I on the other hand was absolutely devastated. I knew it'd be no easy feat but he shot me down completely in such an arrogant manner, that I was angered with the whole experience. I called my other half on the way home, who was just as annoyed and it was actually him that said *"We're going to order you NDT tonight. That's it."*.

You see, in the six months that I'd been on Levothyroxine following official diagnosis of Hashimoto's and hypothyroidism, my partner only saw me decline further and further, and in more ways than one. In his words, I was a shell of who I used to be and I was so depressed that my life was in tatters. I was barely keeping up with work, attending just one day a week out of my usual five, at times. Housework was mounting up and never done and I was just sleeping all the time. When I wasn't sleeping, I was reading up on getting myself better or just plain crying. I had no quality of life, no happiness or youth. I wasn't living, I was just *existing*.

It was m-i-s-e-r-a-b-l-e.

I cannot begin to describe the level of fatigue I experienced, the muscle and joint pain, the brain fog, sensitivity to cold, constipation, depression, anxiety and so much more. Well, you probably know if you're a patient yourself. It's indescribable. The best way I can put it is that it's like having the worst flu of your life, but with other illnesses on top of it and the inability to cope with life's stresses thrown in too. You're just so worn down. I was a mess indeed.

But as I lay on the sofa that night, curled up like a ball trying not to cry anymore from the physical and mental pain that I was in, because I was SO tired of crying, my other half spent countless hours searching for NDT online. Online pharmacies, charities, advocacies, speaking to other thyroid patients etc. all pointing to places where you could source this medication safely yourself. And then with a few clicks, it was done and he turned to me and said *"That's it. It'll be here in a few weeks."*.

I'd already begun reading Stop The Thyroid Madness' website about the use of NDT medication and wanted their book, so we ordered this, which contained all the information I needed to safely dose and use NDT and I began reading this weeks before the medication arrived so that I was clued up on what to do.

Don't get me wrong, I certainly had mixed feelings. I definitely wanted to try NDT since I felt it was the only option out of the misery I was in, unable to work and bed-bound most days. But I was also anxious. I was going to use a medication without a doctor's guidance and this was totally alien to me - I'd never done anything like it before - and friends expressed their concern about it all. *I* was even concerned, but I knew it was my last option. I was suicidal at just twenty-two years old, as I couldn't bear the thought of what the rest of my life would be like if this is how bad I was at twenty-two.

So, by the time it arrived, I had already read my copy of Stop The Thyroid Madness' book and pretty much their whole website, a good few times, which seems to be the leading source on NDT information. My other half also read a lot of it so that he knew what the protocol was and then I began on it, also going in to see my GP and share with him my decision. And this is also where The Invisible Hypothyroidism was born. I setup a WordPress account and wrote my first blog "Starting NDT" where I shared my thoughts and feelings on starting the new medication the next day and then I checked in every week or two with updates on how it was going and any changes in dose, all before my blog actually went live.

You see, I never created The Invisible Hypothyroidism with the intention of becoming a thyroid advocate *or* writer. It was just somewhere to express myself, my thoughts and feelings, struggles and successes, and it wasn't until three and a half months later that I thought *actually, I'm going to share this journey with others,* and I made my blog public, beginning what would be a wonderful and enlightening journey.

## Chapter Recap:

- Although helpful for some, T4-only medication doesn't eliminate symptoms for every person with hypothyroidism.

- A conversion issue is the most common reason for this.

- Other medication options *are* available but doctors are often reluctant to prescribe them due to a lack of knowledge and complicated history.

- Some patients therefore turn to a private prescription or as a very last resort, self-sourcing.

# Chapter 4: When There's Something Else at Play

*"No two people are exactly the same, which means that no two people will heal exactly the same." - Rachel Hill, The Invisible Hypothyroidism*

As well as getting the correct type of thyroid medication for you and the optimal dosage, it's also important to address other issues and factors that can be contributing to you feeling unwell.

I thought for a long while that once I reached my optimal dosage of NDT, with lab results to match, that I would return to the level of health and fitness that I had before. But I didn't. Even with optimal levels, I still had ongoing fatigue, poor stamina, cystic acne and irregular periods, which suggested that I needed to look at other issues and imbalances within my body. I often refer to treating hypothyroidism as piecing together a big jigsaw puzzle. There are often many pieces and these pieces can differ from person to person.

Each person's journey back to good health with hypothyroidism is different and what *you* may need to get there could well be different to myself. And other people.

A lot of research led me to many possible jigsaw puzzle pieces, but I'll sum the big ones up below for you to look in to. This is a particularly large chapter, but that's because there are so many puzzle pieces to mention!

## Leaky Gut

Hippocrates, a Greek Physician often considered to be one of the most outstanding figures in the history of medicine, said *"All disease begins in the gut" and* 2500 years later, we're *just* beginning to understand how right he was.

What's important to know is that poor gut health can suppress thyroid function and trigger Hashimoto's, but low thyroid function can also *lead* to leaky gut, so it works both ways. Various sources including Thyroid Pharmacist Izabella Wentz, state that leaky gut needs to be present to trigger Hashimoto's in the first place, so chances are, most of us have a leaky gut. But what is it? What *am* I on about?!

'Leaky Gut' is used to refer to when the intestinal barrier of the gut becomes permeable from hypothyroidism, infections, food intolerances (especially gluten) or even stress, which then goes on to cause other problems and symptoms. Common symptoms of leaky gut include constipation, wind, bloating, impaired metabolism, ongoing fatigue, mental health struggles, weight gain, a coating on the tongue, a large scalloped tongue, heartburn, acid reflux, bad breath, nutrient malabsorption, skin conditions and more.

The gut assists in converting inactive thyroid hormone T4 to T3, which requires an enzyme called intestinal sulfatase, however this enzyme comes from healthy gut bacteria. Intestinal dysbiosis, something I have experience with myself, is an imbalance between pathogenic and beneficial bacteria in the gut, which can significantly reduce the conversion[20] - just one reason why people with poor gut health may have thyroid symptoms but normal test results. But don't expect your conventional doctor to pay much attention to this. We are in an age where gut health is finally starting to be understood by conventional medicine, as more research is done every week to explore the connection between the gut and rest of the body, but they're still quite a bit behind functional medicine in this topic.

One particular symptom of poor gut health, constipation, can also have knock on effects. It can impair hormone clearance from the body, which causes oestrogen levels to rise. These high oestrogen levels can then decrease the amount of thyroid hormones available[21], making you feel more hypothyroid and fatigued. It's a real catch-22 situation and we know that constipation or non-regular bowel movements are a common symptom of hypothyroidism, too.

Functional medicine also says that any inflammation within the gut can lead or contribute to adrenal fatigue (though it is more accurately referred to as hypothalamic-pituitary axis dysfunction) - something else I have experience with. A response from the adrenal glands in the face of prolonged stress, causing long term adrenal dysfunction. Adrenal fatigue can cause a whole list of symptoms on its own but does also impact thyroid function since they're both part of the endocrine system. More on that soon.

## Candida (Yeast Overgrowth)

Candida is a type of leaky gut where you have an overgrowth of yeast in your body, causing all kinds of issues. And yep, I do indeed have experience with this thyroid jigsaw puzzle piece too.

Yeast exists in the gut naturally and, in the right amount, isn't an issue, but high stress, antibiotics and too much sugar can cause it to thrive and become power hungry. Have hormonal issues? Still feeling fatigued? Stressed a lot? Have any other ongoing symptoms? Please do check for candida. My guess is that you have it.

For me, my usually regular periods started to become massively irregular and could come at any time. At twenty-two, I also began breaking out in severe, cystic acne. I'm not talking a few pimples, I mean that so much of my face was covered in these deep, painful spots that they joined up to cause mountains of pain on my cheeks. Doctors checked for STI's, PCOS and even ran bloods on my sex hormone levels but came up with no answer. I was sure I had an imbalance of too much oestrogen after researching in books and online. It turns out I was right.

A candida overgrowth, often caused by a high sugar diet, high stress levels, anxiety and antibiotic use, is very common in thyroid patients. In my case, dysbiosis had occurred, following extremely high stress levels for years (both mentally and physically), various rounds of antibiotics and a high sugar diet (I've always had an intense sweet tooth). My first appointment with a functional medicine practitioner confirmed the overgrowth but trying to pinpoint when exactly it started was hard, since I'd never gone to the loo regularly enough (just once every 1-2 weeks until I reached my twenties) and it was most likely in place to trigger my Hashimoto's at seventeen years old.

Since being confirmed as having a leaky gut in the form of candida, I've been taking probiotics daily to replenish the good bacteria in my gut, digestive enzymes to help move things along and absorb nutrients from my food properly and oregano oil, a herbal remedy to tame and clear my body of the excess yeast (all with the guidance of my doctor). I've also cut out alcohol and dairy, am following a very low sugar diet, and implementing helpful foods such as anything high in protein, chia seeds, coconut oil, apple cider vinegar, turmeric, cinnamon, flaxseed, hemp oil, oregano and garlic, all to support my gut health and the process of overcoming candida.

For most patients, following this kind of treatment for a few months is long enough to restore the correct balance of yeast and good bacteria in the gut, but for some, it can take longer. It of course also depends on how strictly you're following the advice of your doctor (I see a functional medicine practitioner, since conventional medicine doesn't really recognise leaky gut as an issue to be treated right now) and how severe your case is.

After the balance has been restored, you can often reintroduce more foods, but bearing in mind that you'll need to promote good gut health going forward, so as not to relapse again.

Overcoming a leaky gut and especially candida, can result in much improved energy levels, skin complaints resolving, sex hormones in better balance and even better mental health. It also often resolves or greatly improves high cortisol levels (adrenal fatigue/dysfunction).

## Gluten

'Gluten-free' is a phrase I'm sure you've seen a lot. If you have hypothyroidism, specifically Hashimoto's, it's worth knowing why so many thyroid patients say that being gluten-free helps them.

As already mentioned, it is reported that 90% of people with an underactive thyroid, have the autoimmune disease Hashimoto's Thyroiditis, which attacks the thyroid gland, causing hypothyroidism. A common symptom of this autoimmune disease is gluten sensitivity. But did you know that you could be sensitive to gluten i.e. have it still cause you symptoms or problems, but not be full blown Coeliac?

As hypothyroid patients, it's actually quite likely that we do have a gluten sensitivity due to 'molecular mimicry' as explained in Chapter 2.

You could have had the tests done by your doctor to check for Coeliac Disease, and it come back negative, yet you suffer from symptoms such as:

- Fatigue
- Mood swings/Depression/Anxiety (Research[22] [23] confirms that gluten intolerance can be linked to mental health and mood)
- Brain fog
- Aches and pains
- Joint pain
- Skin issues
- Swinging lab results and feeling hypo then hyper and vice versa
- Poor gut health/leaky gut, also meaning low absorption rate of minerals and vitamins
- Migraines and headaches

**What is The Connection?**

After the introduction to gluten and thyroid disease in Chapter 2, let me now explain in more detail. Gluten is said to trigger the same autoimmune reactions that cause you to have Hashimoto's in the first place, since supposedly, the cells of your thyroid are similar to the molecular structure of gluten, and it confuses your body, increasing inflammation and antibodies as an attack on your thyroid is launched, destroying more thyroid tissue, and so worse/extra hypothyroid symptoms occur. As a result, many Hashimoto's patients eliminate gluten from their diet, and see good results.

Worsening thyroid hormone levels over time as well as swinging test results, are thought to typically be due to the ongoing destruction of your thyroid gland, which obviously causes it to not work properly.

Many thyroid patients try a gluten-free diet and report good results with it and I am one of those. When Italian researchers put subclinical or 'borderline' hypothyroid people with coeliac disease on a gluten-free diet for one-year, thyroid function normalised in 71% of them, with another 19% normalising their thyroid antibodies. The researchers concluded that in some cases, a gluten-free diet may single-handedly reverse the abnormality[24]. *The Effect of Gluten-Free Diet on Thyroid Autoimmunity in Drug-Naive Women With Hashimoto's Thyroiditis: A Pilot Study* also concluded that their results suggested a gluten-free diet may bring clinical benefits to women with Hashimoto's[25].

Consuming gluten can also reportedly lead to leaky gut, where holes form in the gut lining and when food is ingested, like gluten in this instance, it allows small particles to leak into the bloodstream, leading to symptoms of gluten sensitivity like those listed above. In the idea of molecular mimicry, the immune system sees these particles as foreign entities, creates antibodies and mounts an attack not only on the foreign protein, gluten, but also on thyroid tissue because of its close resemblance to gluten. Eek!

If you often have low levels in vitamins (B12, D, Iron etc.), it could well indicate Hashimoto's and/or damage to the gut caused by consuming gluten.

Dr Datis Kharrazian has also commented that having Hashimoto's and consuming gluten can cause inflammation in the brain, leading to brain fog.

## Joint and Muscle Aches

Gluten caused inflammation can reportedly cause joint and muscle pain in some people.[26]

The Arthritis Foundation has also published information regarding the link between gluten sensitivity, joint pain, and arthritis conditions. [27]

If you think you could be sensitive or allergic to gluten, or are just interested in giving gluten-free a try to see if it helps your fatigue, aches and pains, etc. try eliminating it from your diet for at least a few months and keep a log of how you feel. You should also ideally retest your thyroid antibodies, TPOAB and TGAB, to see if they come down. This will give you an idea of whether a gluten-free diet is helping to control your thyroid condition.

Being a total foodie and protective over my food, I was reluctant to go gluten-free for quite a while. My first attempt at it was also quite half-hearted and I caved in after not so long. The second time around, I wanted to take it more seriously and haven't looked back since. You soon adapt and don't even really think about it. For me, it's drastically helped my cystic acne, heart palpitations, sleep, constipation, wind and more. I'll never go back. On the other hand, though, I've heard from many people with Hashimoto's and hypothyroidism who feel no difference being gluten-free whatsoever. Like I said previously, we have to figure out what works for us in our own situation as every individual is just that: *individual.*

## Adrenal Fatigue

Adrenal fatigue (though it is more accurately referred to as hypothalamic-pituitary axis dysfunction) is a condition not widely recognised by mainstream medicine yet, though I believe it's only a matter of time until it is. It just makes so much sense.

The adrenal glands, which sit atop the kidneys, are responsible for producing hormones in relation to stress and the one concerned in adrenal fatigue in cortisol. Now, there are two recognised conditions in conventional medicine, in association with extreme dysfunctioning of the adrenal glands: Addison's Disease, which is a long term condition whereby the adrenal glands do not produce enough cortisol and Cushing's, which is the opposite - where the adrenals produce often dangerously high levels of the hormone.

'Adrenal fatigue' or hypothalamic-pituitary axis dysfunction, is a condition well recognised within functional medicine, where the adrenal glands produce too much or too little cortisol, though not to the extent of Cushing's Disease or Addison's Disease, but abnormal enough that it causes symptoms and issues all the same. It works on the idea that there is a scale rather than just extremes.

Adrenal fatigue can include elevated, lowered or mixed levels of cortisol, without it being the full blown condition of one of those two extremes. This condition is very real. Thousands of people report symptoms and problems with adrenal issues (high, low or mixed cortisol levels) and then state they're gone once cortisol levels gave returned to ideal numbers.

The below symptoms have been collated from various adrenal fatigue information websites and patients:

- Struggling to fall asleep at night, or waking up a few hours after you do
- Feeling more tired in the morning
- Having a mid-afternoon 'slump'
- Feeling over-emotional
- Having anxiety
- Having ongoing fatigue that affects your day to day life
- Often wanting to be alone
- Unable to tolerate stress
- Hot flashes/sweats
- Jumping or feeling irritable at loud noises
- Being a bit sensitive and taking things to heart more so than you used to
- Being on thyroid medication for a while and still not feeling better

- Having been hypothyroid for several years *before* being diagnosed
- Having been through chronic emotional, mental or biological stress
- Craving for salty foods
- A weakened immune system
- Asthma, allergies or respiratory complaints
- Dark circles under the eyes
- Dizziness
- Mental fog
- Changes in bowel movements
- Sudden sensitivities to certain foods, like gluten or dairy
- Dizziness, imbalance, collapsing and blacking out
- Dry mouth
- Joint pain
- Weight gain or weight loss
- Low libido
- Coldness in hands/feet
- Strong cravings for sugar/salt
- Leaky gut, GERD, GORD, acid reflux
- Dry skin
- Extreme tiredness after exercise
- Loss of muscle tone
- Lower back pain
- Numbness in your fingers / Poor circulation

- Unable to fall asleep despite being tired
- Heart palpitations
- Low thyroid function
- Feeling of hypoglycaemia (low blood sugar though test results are normal
- Hair falling out
- Muscle pain of unknown reason
- Inability to concentrate or focus
- Short of breath even though breathing is fine
- Legs that feel heavy at times
- Chronic Fatigue Syndrome unimproved with conventional help
- Fibromyalgia unresolved after conventional help
- Irregular menstrual cycles

The adrenal glands are part of the endocrine system, just like the thyroid. They handle many hormones that are important for a lot of bodily processes, such as handling stress, and this is where cortisol comes in.

According to James Wilson's book *Adrenal Fatigue: The 21st Century Stress Syndrome*, the adrenals first respond to stress by providing you with extra cortisol, but the body can only keep up with high cortisol for so long. So after this, the cortisol starts to fall, leading to low cortisol. In between this, you could experience combined highs and lows.

You could have high, low or combined high and low cortisol causing these symptoms and thus adrenal fatigue. Cortisol has a variety of important functions, including:

the metabolism of carbohydrates, proteins and fats, affecting blood sugar levels in your blood, helping reduce inflammation and helping you deal with stress. The latter is especially huge.

As I write this book, I am suffering from adrenal issues (high cortisol), after being left hypothyroid for too long without treatment, and then being held to Levothyroxine when I did get treatment, which wasn't the right medication for me. I arranged for a saliva test to be done privately (a 24 hour, four point saliva test). When I got the results back, they showed that my cortisol was elevated 24 hours a day, indicating adrenal dysfunction and a cause for many of my ongoing symptoms; mainly fatigue.

In terms of exercising, Dr Sara Gottfried explains in her book *The Hormone Cure*, that a sign of adrenal issues can even include trying to exercise, only to find you crash, feeling light-headed and faint. This is due to cortisol being part of the glucocorticoid family, a substance that raises your glucose level. It is cortisol's job to give you the energy you need. When you have this reaction to exercise, it's a sign you've used up your main energy supply as you're perhaps low on cortisol and so don't have enough ready to use.

So, adrenal fatigue could be caused by low, high or combined low and high cortisol. What are the stages of adrenal fatigue?

**High Cortisol - Stage One**

High cortisol has very similar symptoms to low cortisol, and is usually the first stage of adrenal fatigue. If you can catch it while it's still at this stage then you may have an easier time addressing and correcting the adrenal fatigue.

High bedtime cortisol can cause disruption of your sleep pattern, resulting in problems falling asleep, or staying asleep, so this could be a key sign also.

## Combined High and Low Cortisol - Stage Two

This stage is thought to come between high cortisol and low cortisol, when the adrenals cannot keep up with high cortisol any longer, and so it starts to drop at certain points.

## Low Cortisol - Stage Three

This is not the same as the disease called Addison's, low cortisol is actually a long-term situation where, though your adrenals may still work, they are either out-of-sync or inhibited. As explained above, this happens when they first produced elevated cortisol, then combined highs and lows of cortisol, and then low cortisol.

## But How Do I Fix My Adrenals?

Usually lifestyle and dietary changes need to be made, in order to recover from adrenal issues, but it's very much individual to each person. Certain adaptogenic herbs can also help in addition to these changes. Lots of information on this can be found in James Wilson's book but I'd also recommend consulting a medical practitioner who fully recognises adrenal dysfunction, such as a functional doctor, naturopath etc. as having their guidance and unearthing root causes is often crucial.

Issues such as a sex hormone imbalances, leaky gut, high thyroid antibodies, diet and food sensitivities are often the root cause behind 'adrenal fatigue' but you have to figure out what it is for *you*. All of them were behind mine!

## Vitamin Levels and Supplementing

There are certain supplements that support thyroid function as they work to maintain optimal levels, where most patients tend to state they feel best. As recovering from hypothyroidism is like piecing together a jigsaw puzzle, it is important to consider other possible problems beside your thyroid condition, such as low vitamin levels and other health conditions, in getting you back to good health.

I would always recommend consulting your doctor, pharmacist, a medical professional etc. before making any changes to your health regimen as it can be dangerous if you take supplements and already have high/sufficient levels. This is especially true for pregnant women who should always speak to a medical professional before making any changes. Only take supplements to maintain or replace vitamins and minerals you are sure you are deficient in.

If you're gluten  or dairy free, or have any other restrictions, do also always check that all supplements you take are free of the offending substance, too.

Most vitamins can be tested via doctor ordered tests to learn your levels, but you can also order tests yourself online. I cannot state personalised dosages for you as it depends on your own needs. Please establish these with a medical professional's guidance.

## B Vitamins/B-Complex

B1, B2, B3, B6 and B12 can help tiredness, fatigue, metabolic function and promote good adrenal health and function. Vitamin B12 and folic acid are both important for energy and heart protection and folic acid is also good for preventing neural tube defects in a developing baby. It is also needed in order to make TSH. B3 is needed to keep all the body's cells (including the endocrine glands) in efficient working order. People with hypothyroidism tend to struggle to absorb B12, of which a lack can cause mental illness, various neurological disorders, neuralgia, neuritis and bursitis. A leaky gut and poor gut health could well be behind why so many of us have low levels. Vegan and vegetarian diets also pose more risk of low B vitamins and taking excessive amounts of Vitamin C can also decrease the availability of Vitamin B12.

## Iron

For many thyroid patients, low iron levels cause fatigue, depression, aches and pains and lack of stamina. Always have your levels tested before taking a supplement as taking extra iron can be dangerous. Bisglycinate is a popular type of iron as it doesn't cause stomach issues or constipation. Taking iron supplements with Vitamin C can increase absorption significantly. It is worth bearing in mind that as hypothyroidism mainly affects women, many thyroid patients will have low levels of iron/ferritin due to period issues such as heavy or long periods.

## Vitamin E

An antioxidant, Vitamin E is a fat-soluble vitamin important for many processes in the body, including producing TSH and maintaining healthy skin.

## Selenium

Selenium helps the conversion of T4 to T3. Without it, T3 cannot be produced in the right amounts, and organs will function as if they are hypothyroid even though blood test levels are 'normal'. It is also vital for the immune system and reproduction. With low selenium levels, you could have symptoms such as brain fog and decreased cognitive functions, as well as a lack of energy. You could also have low Free T3 as a sign that selenium is low or deficient, causing not enough T4 to T3 conversion. It is also an antioxidant. It is also reported to lower thyroid antibodies[28], helping to manage Hashimoto's more effectively.

## Vitamin C

Essential for the immune system and adrenals, the adrenal glands contain the highest concentration of Vitamin C in the body. This famous vitamin plays a crucial role in both the adrenal cortex and adrenal medulla, which are responsible for responding to stress.

## Iodine

A controversial one, many say you should only supplement it if you are definitely low in it, as it can do more harm than good if not. Sufficient iodine is needed to make thyroid hormone T4. Many thyroid patients state they found they indeed needed iodine after doing iodine testing. Iodine is required for the normal process of metabolisation of cells and is needed for a normally functioning thyroid – the production mechanisms of thyroid hormones. You can present with a goitre if you're lacking in iodine due to thyroid cells enlarging.

## Vitamin D3 and A

Good for joints and addressing fatigue, a deficiency in Vitamin A or D can also stop T3 from correcting your metabolic rate and leave you with low energy, cold intolerance and weight gain. Low levels of Vitamin D can cause depression, back pain, joint pain and stiffness, fatigue and poor immune system function. Vitamin A must be accompanied by protein to make it available to the body, so if you are on a low protein diet, you may be deficient in this. If you are low on Vitamin A, your ability to produce TSH is limited. This vitamin is required by the body to convert T4 to T3. Vitamin D has also been shown to lower antibodies.[29]

Caution is required with supplementing Vitamin A if trying to conceive or pregnant, due to potential toxicity levels. Vitamin D has also been shown to lower thyroid antibodies.

## Vitamin K2

You should always take Vitamin D3 with K2. K2 regulates calcium in the blood, so combining Vitamin K2 with Vitamin D3 is highly recommended because of the synergy between the two vitamins. Research shows a slower progression of calcification in those taking both Vitamin K2 and vitamin D3 compared to those taking Vitamin D3 alone.

## Zinc

Zinc is required for the body to make TSH. Research has shown that both hypothyroidism and hyperthyroidism can result in zinc deficiency and it also plays a role in the proper functioning of the immune system. Zinc is also great for gut health.

## Fish Oil/Omega 3/Cod Liver Oil

Cod Liver Oil is one of the best sources of Omega 3 fatty acids (EPA and DHA) and contains relatively high amounts of Vitamin A and D. Good for lowering high blood pressure, reducing risk of osteoarthritis and maintaining joint and bone health.

## Magnesium

Magnesium is needed in order to make TSH and for the conversion of T4 into T3. It seems that a diet high in refined food and caffeine will encourage magnesium loss. Magnesium can also help cramps and aches and pains.

## Probiotic

Probiotics provide 'good' gut bacteria that can improve overall gut health and strengthen the immune system.

# Other Conditions Which Often Come Hand in Hand With Hypothyroidism

Soon after my diagnosis of autoimmune hypothyroidism, I learnt that it was also important to address other health conditions that often go hand in hand with them. As well as leaky gut, gluten sensitivity, 'adrenal fatigue' and the vitamin deficiencies already mentioned, it's also worth being aware of the below.

## Mental Health Conditions

Not all thyroid patients experience mental health difficulties but a fair few do.

The symptoms of hypothyroidism can cause, be linked to, or have an effect on our mental health, such as depression and anxiety. I have had both of these mental health conditions. This is linked to the thyroid hormone T3, which many hypothyroid patients do not have a lot of.

In fact, thyroid patients of all ages may be labelled with psychiatric issues such as mental health issues, when they are actually due to hormonal insufficiencies such as 'adrenal fatigue'. In one study[30], it was concluded that by correcting the underlying hormonal imbalance, many patients' mental health improved, with some patients having a *total* reversal of psychiatric symptoms.

And according to Thyroid UK's survey in 2015[31], over 50% of the hypothyroidism patients who took part in the survey also had depression. That's more than half and of those taking antidepressants, 47% saw no difference. Why? Most likely because the underlying problem, being the poorly treated thyroid condition, missed vitamin deficiencies or possibly even adrenal fatigue, hadn't been addressed.

So as not to confuse the two conditions and their symptoms, let's make it clear that there *are* some symptoms of depression that are the same as those for hypothyroidism, such as:

- Low mood
- Being slow in speech and/or movement
- Constipation
- Feeling more tired than normal

But equally, there are some **that are not present** in depression, such as:

- Thinning of eyebrows
- A puffy face
- Overwhelming fatigue
- Dry skin
- Hoarse voice
- Muscle weakness
- Raised blood pressure
- Raised cholesterol

These are *physical* symptoms, and not caused by something mental, but something *physically* wrong. They could well be a sign that the thyroid patient isn't adequately treated on their thyroid medication and this needs investigating.

The link between depression and thyroid problems is thought to involve T3, one of the hormones a healthy thyroid should be producing. Unfortunately, 99% of the time doctors in the UK especially will only prescribe T4-only medications (like Levothyroxine) for hypothyroidism (and it doesn't seem much different in other countries either) so we're relying on our bodies to convert some of that in to the T3.

## Taking Medication for Mental Health Conditions Isn't Wrong

Antidepressants or anti-anxiety medications can be a great help to many people and it is important to not feed the stigma that taking them is in any way 'wrong'. I am not anti-medication, but I am pro-informed decision, which means making sure those that who are thyroid patients also experiencing mental health conditions, know that addressing their endocrine health fully may well resolve their mental health complaints.

I have taken various types of antidepressants myself in the past. However, none helped me at all, which is perhaps a sign that it was due to a physical imbalance of thyroid hormone. Especially as my mental health hugely improved when optimally medicated for hypothyroidism.

## Hypothyroidism and Your Mental Health

Having low Free T3 is a likely cause for depression, mood swings, anxiety etc. when on T4-only medicine, as once this is treated with direct T3, it often improves greatly. This was certainly true for me. When I switched from T4-only Levothyroxine to NDT, which contains direct T3, my anxiety, depression and over-emotional tendencies improved quickly.

T3 has an important role in the health and optimal functioning of your brain, including: your cognitive function, ability to concentrate, mood, memory and attention span and emotions and ability to cope with life's stresses.

T3 interacts with brain receptors and makes the brain more sensitive to chemicals such as serotonin and norepinephrine, which affects your alertness, memory, mood and emotion.

So if your doctor failed to check a full thyroid panel, when you complained about feeling low and depressed, you may have mental health issues caused by an inadequately treated thyroid problem.

If you have had a full panel conducted, be sure to check that they fall within optimal levels; a TSH below 2, Free T3 within the top quarter of the range and a Free T4 mid-range or higher.

## Hashimoto's and Your Mental Health

Hashimoto's, prevalent in about 90% of us with hypothyroidism, is reported to cause swings of TSH due to ongoing destruction of the thyroid gland, with hyperthyroid and hypothyroid symptoms to match. Hyperthyroid symptoms can include a sudden 'burst' of energy, anxiety, irritability and disturbed sleep, whilst hypothyroidism often causes fatigue, slowness and depression. Do those swinging symptoms remind you of anything? Bipolar disorder perhaps?

Also known as manic depression, it could well be suggested that some bipolar diagnoses are actually masking Hashimoto's cases, where patients swing between hypo and hyper symptoms, as the thyroid is attacked and destroyed, and thyroid hormone is released into the bloodstream in waves. Indeed, I've had thyroid patients contact me to say they spent time in a mental health hospital or a loved one did, for psychiatric issues that were later discovered to be down to untreated hypothyroidism or Hashimoto's.

The 2002 study *High Rate of Autoimmune Thyroiditis in Bipolar Disorder: Lack of Association with Lithium Exposure*[32], found that Hashimoto's antibodies were more prevalent in a sample of outpatients with bipolar disorder (28%), in comparison to a control group (3-18%). However, what complicates things is that bipolar patients are often treated with Lithium, a drug well-recognised to cause hypothyroidism and trigger Hashimoto's. So, was the thyroid condition there first, or did the lithium cause it?

Getting your Hashimoto's well controlled may help with mental health.

## Adrenals and Your Mental Health

Adrenal issues could also be causing or contributing to a thyroid patient's depression, anxiety and emotional health. Abnormal cortisol levels, which are very common among hypothyroid patients, can result in cell receptors failing to properly receive T3 from the blood, which can explain why you may have some behaviour and symptoms typical of depression and continued hypothyroid symptoms, including:

- Wanting to be alone
- Unable to tolerate stress
- Jumping or feeling irritable at loud noises
- Emotional ups and downs
- Anxiety
- Being a bit sensitive and taking things to heart more so than you used to.

So, if you have depression, anxiety, bipolar disorder etc. or you've been diagnosed with another mental health condition, and also have thyroid or adrenal problems, or suspect you do, explore the above ideas and check they're all in line. You may just find checking your thyroid, vitamin levels and cortisol levels help you, and ensuring you have adequate Free T3 levels, like adding T3 did for me.

Although we must stress here that taking medication for mental health conditions, such as antidepressants, isn't *wrong*, by piling on more medication without addressing the root cause, it's not helping us in the long-term. Doctors need to stop giving us more and more medications that we may not actually need, and instead concentrate on making sure our endocrine health is optimised in the first place. Is it better for someone to be put on an unnecessary antidepressant or have the underlying cause addressed?

## Goitres and Nodules

Have you ever noticed that your neck seems enlarged or been told it 'sticks out'? Have you experienced hoarseness? Do you struggle to swallow or feel a lump in your throat? You could have an enlarged thyroid gland, also called a goitre, or a nodule. It can be slight or very noticeable and is caused when your thyroid over exerts itself.

If you have Hashimoto's then this can cause the thyroid to swell from inflammation. It is generally believed that treating your Hashimoto's successfully decreases the inflammation and size of the goitre.

However, another reason for enlargement could be nodules on the thyroid. A nodule is a swelling or lump, which can be a solid or liquid filled cyst or mass. The cause for them is pretty unknown, but patients can see these abnormal growths from being left undiagnosed or from the use of T4-only medication like Levothyroxine, which often leave thyroid levels below optimal. These causes suggest that inadequate treatment and management of the thyroid can lead to nodules. More than 90% of all thyroid nodules are usually benign[33]. Only a very small percentage of these are cancerous, so try not to worry. However, you will require a thorough examination from a doctor and an ultrasound to look in to it further.

Iodine deficiency can also cause nodules, but it's important to not supplement with iodine unless you know you are deficient. Dr Datis Kharrazian also suggests that it can aggravate Hashimoto's. Eating a lot of goitrogenic foods is said to negatively affect iodine use by the thyroid, too.

## Thyroid Cancer

And although I don't by any means want to frighten any of you, it is important to state that cancer of the thyroid gland is another, albeit small possibility for a goitre or nodule, and is diagnosed by doing a fine needle biopsy.

You can check your thyroid by following the below steps:

1. Stand in front of a mirror, removing anything that doesn't give you a clear view of your neck, like jumpers and scarves.
2. Stretch your neck back, with your chin pointing towards the ceiling.
3. Feel where your thyroid is, and around it, very gently, to see if you can feel any enlargement, lumps or pain.
4. Closely look at your neck too, looking for any enlargement or lumpiness. Swallowing some water might help to highlight anything.
5. If you think you can feel something not quite right, like any enlargement, tenderness (besides the uncomfortable feeling of touching your neck area) or lumps, you should see a doctor as soon as possible to be assessed.

## Graves' Disease

Like Hashimoto's, your thyroid can become enlarged due to having Graves' Disease, another autoimmune disease. With Graves', your thyroid hormones increase and increase, and your TSH gets progressively lower as you become more hyperthyroid. You'll need to get this properly treated to bring the size of an enlarged thyroid gland down.

It is possible to have both Graves' and Hashimoto's, although quite rare.

## Subacute Thyroiditis

Subacute thyroiditis is a rare condition and is thought to be caused by a viral infection, as it often occurs after one, such as mumps, flu or a cold. The first signs are soreness and tenderness in the area of the thyroid gland, and sometimes pain spreading to other parts of the neck, ears or jaw, with symptoms of hyperthyroidism or, later, hyperthyroidism. It may cause your neck to feel sore.

At the end of the day, if your thyroid or neck looks enlarged, you really ought to explore why, and I strongly suggest having a doctor examine it as soon as you notice.

## PCOS (Polycystic Ovary Syndrome)

On average, women with PCOS tend to have higher TSH levels and be subclinically (borderline) hypothyroid when compared to controls of the same age without PCOS. Hypothyroidism, and in particular, Hashimoto's thyroiditis, is more common in women with PCOS than in the general population. So, hypothyroidism and PCOS are often seem together.

PCOS symptoms of irregular periods, non-ovulation, high levels of male hormones in the body (excess androgen) which can lead to excess facial and body hair, failure to conceive, weight gain, acne and hair loss from the scalp can all be mixed up with symptoms of a thyroid condition such as Hashimoto's and hypothyroidism, so knowing where one condition starts and another ends can be tricky.

## Migraines

Many thyroid patients also experience migraines. A migraine is more than a regular headache. They can be debilitating and are often not helped by regular painkillers such as paracetamol or ibuprofen. The pain often felt behind one eye or on one side of the head is a deep, distracting throbbing that is often accompanied by nausea, disturbed vision, sensitivity to light, sound and even movement. Some people also feel dizzy and faint with a migraine.

Research has suggested a connection between thyroid disease and migraines. One study, including more than 8,400 participants observed over twenty years, suggested that those with a pre-existing headache disorder such as migraine, have a 21% greater risk of developing hypothyroidism. Also, very interestingly, those already experiencing migraines are a whopping 41% more likely to become hypothyroid.[34]

## Other Conditions Hypothyroidism Can Masquerade As

There are some conditions that can coexist with hypothyroidism, particularly from a poorly managed underactive thyroid. A lot of these result from low levels of Free T4 and Free T3, despite being on thyroid medication. Don't let your list of diagnoses grow due to being non-optimal on thyroid medication.

## Infertility and Pregnancy Complications

Thyroid function and fertility are closely linked. Abnormal thyroid levels can lead to miscarriage, preeclampsia, anaemia, stillbirth and the baby developing congenital hypothyroidism itself, yet many doctors don't think to check thyroid hormone levels when pregnancy or fertility issues occur.

Thyroid hormones directly affect the uterine lining, causing infertility or miscarriages to occur when they are abnormal. As well as complications during pregnancy, some women with low thyroid levels may even struggle to fall pregnant at all. Hormones TSH and TRH are ramped up when thyroid hormones such as Free T3 and Free T4 fall too low; TRH to stimulate the pituitary gland to release TSH, which *then* instructs the thyroid gland to release more thyroid hormones T3 and T4.

Infertility can therefore occur when TRH, which is also responsible for stimulating the pituitary gland to release prolactin, causes the increased prolactin to interfere with the ovulation process, when thyroid hormones are low. The increased prolactin levels (prolactin is also important for promoting lactation) can prevent the ovaries from releasing an egg each month, which makes it more difficult to conceive.

I am also noticing more and more women with sex hormone issues such as oestrogen dominance, which can affect cycles and ovulation. Since the thyroid, pituitary and ovaries are all part of the endocrine system, it's not difficult to understand why having problems with one of these, may also mean having issues with another.

Therefore, ensuring your thyroid levels, TSH, Free T3 and Free T4, are all optimal is crucial when trying to conceive, as is checking your ratio of oestrogen to progesterone.

Most women require an increase in thyroid medication when pregnant, to support the developing baby and failure to properly maintain adequate thyroid levels whilst pregnant can result in complications such as miscarriage, preeclampsia, anaemia, stillbirth and the baby developing congenital hypothyroidism itself. So, it's very important to be tested regularly, often every 6-12 weeks, throughout your pregnancy. Adjustments to your medication should then be made accordingly.

## Oestrogen Dominance

I'm one thyroid patient who, after years on the combined contraceptive pill, with period issues such as menorrhagia and irregularity as well as my thyroid issues, found out that I had oestrogen dominance; where the balance of oestrogen to progesterone is very 'off'.

For me, this presented not only with those period issues, but also with severe cystic acne, adrenal fatigue, oily skin, PMS and more. Endometriosis, decreased sex drive, struggling to conceive, PCOS, cervical dysplasia, breast cancer, uterine fibroids and weight gain can also be signs.

The link between oestrogen dominance and hypothyroidism is hard to miss, considering that for every nine or ten women that suffer from hypothyroidism, only one man does. We also know that big hormonal shifts in a woman's body, such as pregnancy or the menopause, can bring hypothyroidism to surface. Many functional medicine practitioners are now blaming oestrogen dominance for the cause of some hypothyroidism cases, as a non-autoimmune cause on its own, but also as a trigger for the autoimmune version of hypothyroidism: Hashimoto's Thyroiditis.

Oestrogen is primarily produced by the ovaries and is responsible for the growth of the uterine lining during the first half of your cycle. Day one of your cycle is the first day of your period. Progesterone is produced by the ovaries as well and its primary role is to prepare the uterus for conception. Both hormones are present throughout the whole cycle but in different amounts depending on where in your cycle you are. Oestrogen dominates the first half and progesterone dominates the second.

Many of us with hypothyroidism have this hormonal imbalance, since the endocrine system is such a delicate dance of various hormones and when one part of that system (the hypothalamus, pituitary, thyroid, parathyroids, adrenals, pineal gland, reproductive organs, pancreas) goes awry, it can have a knock-on effect to others. We already know that many of us have adrenal dysfunction anyway, so it's well worth investigating.

To check if you have oestrogen dominance, you can test your sex hormone levels, testing your progesterone at its peak, around day 21 of your cycle (this may differ or be difficult to predict if you have an irregular cycle), and oestrogen on cycle days 3-5. Testosterone can be tested at any time during the month and checking FSH is also often beneficial. These test results should be able to indicate whether you have an imbalance in your ratio of oestrogen to progesterone, but any symptoms of oestrogen dominance form part of the diagnosis.

## So, what can you do to avoid or combat oestrogen dominance?

First of all, there are some simple changes you can make and things to be aware of. You should ensure that you're eating plenty of fibre and that your bowels are moving often enough so as to support clearance of 'old' oestrogen from the body. Bowel movements of once or twice a day are what you should be aiming for, so eat plenty of fibre rich food (though not close to taking your thyroid medication or it can affect absorption), begin your day with half a lemon squeezed in to some hot water for a drink and start there. After that, if you still have no joy then please do explore leaky gut and digestive enzymes etc. to get your digestive system and bowels working happily. Magnesium supplementation can also aid regular bowel movements.

There is some belief that eating meat and other products of animals can contribute to high oestrogen levels since they contain hormones from the animal itself, so sourcing protein from other places instead of relying on these products entirely may help to lower levels somewhat. But the boat is still out on that one.

Look for BPA-free water bottles, storage containers and minimise exposure through cosmetics and other household products and avoid using hormonal contraceptives, which inevitably upset the oestrogen-progesterone balance and even when you come off them, can take years to correct (like me).

## Avoid Stress

Avoiding stress is easier said than done, I know, but stress is linked to sex hormone levels very delicately. When a person is stressed, the adrenal glands pump out extra cortisol. When this becomes chronic, it disrupts the normal circadian rhythm and the stress response of the Hypothalamus-Pituitary-Adrenal axis. Eventually, the adrenals start to run low on cortisol and begin 'stealing' progesterone to convert in to more cortisol, depleting levels even further, increasing the imbalance between progesterone and oestrogen.

This stress and pressure can then inhibit the liver from converting thyroid hormone T4 (the storage hormone) to T3 (the active hormone), which contributes to us feeling like rubbish and can also prevent it from detoxifying the excess oestrogen. When this happens, the oestrogen can start to build up in tissues and cause oestrogen levels to rise even further.

Work to find what helps you destress and feel calm. Whether that's long walks, sitting in nature, reading, music or yoga.

## Consider Coming Off Hormonal Contraceptives

These medications will not help your hormonal imbalances but instead worsen it.

What can be frustrating is that whilst conventional medicine recognises that increased oestrogen levels can lead to increased chances of fibroids and breast cancer for example, they don't typically look to address the issue directly, looking at the body and endocrine system as a whole. If you've attempted to address oestrogen dominance yourself and aren't having much luck, I strongly recommend seeking out a naturopathic or functional doctor. Doing so has been a godsend for me.

## Period Problems

Along with many of the other symptoms of hypothyroidism, menstrual issues are a common one. Thyroid hormone is needed for pretty much every function and cell in the body so when you're hypothyroid, many processes — including your menstrual cycle — can be affected.

Heavy periods, painful periods, irregular periods, short cycles, delayed periods etc. can all be affected by non-optimal thyroid hormone levels, as well as adrenal issues and oestrogen dominance.

## Low Sex Drive

A low or absent libido is much more common that you think. The thyroid gland is responsible for producing hormones that are needed for every cell and function in our body. They're needed for regulating metabolism, heart rate, temperature (hands up, who's cold a lot of the time?) and blood pressure. They even affect our immune system and sex drive.

To recap on what I've already said about the active thyroid hormone T3: I specify it as being the active hormone since T4, the storage hormone, must be converted into T3, and it's the T3 that we need in order to function well, have energy, a good functioning metabolism and healthy sex drive, but many of us struggle with the conversion process. And with hypothyroidism, when Free

T3 is low, the metabolism is slowed down, which means the reproductive organs can slow down as well.

T3 just so happens to be vital in the functioning of both the ovaries and testes, whereby too little available T3 can cause your sex drive to go out of business and diminish. Remember how I said thyroid hormones are needed for every function and every cell? Yep, even sexual functions and arousal.

And we also know that low thyroid hormones can also cause us to feel low in mood, irritable, overly-emotional, fatigued beyond words and achy. Would you always want to have sex when you feel so rubbish?

Here is an analogy taken from the book: *You, Me and Hypothyroidism: When Someone You Love Has Hypothyroidism:*

*"Imagine someone has cooked you your favourite meal. It has everything you could possibly imagine. It's perfect; the best sirloin steak, the best thin crust pizza, your favourite curry. It's got everything, every possible accompaniment, every side order and your favourite drink to wash it all down with. Except, you're not hungry because you feel sick. You'd love to demolish the entire thing, but can't. It doesn't appeal to you at all. No matter how much you'd like to eat it, you have no appetite and feel so ill. That is what having a low libido can feel like. It's not a case of desire, it's a case of situation. When a chronic illness can make you feel ill every day, sex may not be the top of your priorities."*

As well as thyroid hormones, your adrenal hormones can also be involved. They are involved in the synthesis of

DHEA, testosterone, aldosterone, oestrogen and progesterone, other important hormones. Especially important to your libido and all of these share the same precursor, pregnenolone.

The link between your libido and adrenals occurs here. When adrenal dysfunction exists in the form of high cortisol, it can start to 'steal' more progesterone than is ideal, as it's the precursor to cortisol, in order to produce more cortisol and keep up high levels. This can lead to a sex hormone imbalance, where the ratio of oestrogen to progesterone is very off.

If you have an hypothyroidism, and experience a lack of interest in sex, experience erectile dysfunction or related issues, it's crucial that you have a full thyroid panel tested, to include TSH, Free T4 and that all important Free T3. It would also be worth looking into your adrenals, Reverse T3, sex hormone levels - namely oestrogen, progesterone and testosterone, since abnormal levels in these can also cause a lack of interest in sexual behaviour, but also irregular periods, PMS and tension and irritability with your partner. Perhaps it even annoys you when they suggest sex.

The good news is that when low thyroid hormone levels are corrected, as well as sex hormone levels if applicable, the result is often a return to all bodily functions and processes, including your libido.

**Heart Problems**

Inadequately treated hypothyroidism can affect the health of your heart[35], such as an increase in developing heart disease, and "bad" cholesterol, with high and low blood pressure also. Due to an increase in "bad" cholesterol with many thyroid patients, it can therefore also lead to a hardening of the arteries, which increases your risk of heart attacks and strokes.

I had high blood pressure before my thyroid was properly treated, but also addressing my adrenal fatigue was key in correcting this. The thoughts of heart attacks and strokes are too scary to dismiss.

## Hypoglycaemia

Also known as low blood sugar, it is linked to adrenal health, so having adrenal dysfunction increases your chances of having this. When your blood sugar levels drop below normal, your adrenal glands respond by secreting more cortisol. I've covered this some more in Chapter 2.

## Low Stomach Acid

Stomach acid is needed in the body to break down food and get rid of bad bacteria. It is made as and when you eat, but many hypothyroid patients have low stomach acid, which leads to GORD, GERD, acid reflux, heartburn, indigestion, acid regurgitation, difficulty swallowing, chest pain/discomfort, cough and even hoarseness. You may even feel very full and tired after eating.

As you get older, your levels of stomach acid can decrease, but many hypothyroid patients are surprised to learn that their acid reflux can be related to a poorly treated underactive thyroid, hypothyroidism or Hashimoto's. In fact, Studies have found that people with hypothyroidism (and especially Hashimoto's) often have low stomach acid. Low thyroid hormone levels are often behind it, or leaky gut issues.

## Myxoedema Coma

This is a loss of brain function as a result of longstanding, severely low levels of thyroid hormones. It is considered a life-threatening complication of hypothyroidism but very, very rare these days. If you stop taking your thyroid medication long term, you put yourself at risk for this.

## Fibromyalgia

Although many thyroid patients are told they also have fibromyalgia, a separate condition to their hypothyroidism, and although it *can* be, it may actually be a symptom of a poorly treated thyroid condition. Dr Barry Durrant-Peatfield covers this in his book, *Your Thyroid and how to keep it healthy.. The Great Thyroid Scandal and How to Survive it.*

I've heard many patients say that once they were able to get out of their hypothyroid state, going by a full thyroid panel and raising Free T3 especially to optimal, their fibromyalgia improved or went away altogether.

## Muscle and Joint Pain

Muscle and joint pain, stiffness, cramping and spasming are well reported amongst thyroid patients. Muscle and joint pain caused by hypothyroidism is known as hypothyroid myopathy, and can occur all over the body, though most commonly in the legs, feet, arms, hands and back, ranging from mild to severe.

It also includes cramping, stiffness and weakness, but hypothyroid myopathy can also lead to carpal tunnel syndrome or frozen shoulder.

These symptoms are often caused by thyroid levels being below optimal, low magnesium levels, low Vitamin D levels or even adrenal issues. Therefore, ensuring that all your thyroid levels are optimal, supplementing magnesium, Vitamin D or using Epsom salts for baths/foot soaks and exploring whether you have adrenal fatigue and subsequently treating it, could help you resolve the symptoms. High Reverse T3 or low Free T3 levels in particular should be checked for.

Fluid retention, another somewhat common hypothyroid symptom, can cause pain, too. It's most often seen around the ankles and feet and worsens with physical activity. This is also often solved with optimal thyroid and vitamin levels.

Magnesium spray is popular if you prefer to not add another supplement or tablet to your daily regimen and acupuncture has been helpful to some thyroid patients, too.

Low Vitamin D levels can especially cause joint stiffness and pain, so ensuring you're not low or deficient in it is key too.

## Chronic Fatigue Syndrome/ME

Another condition I have been diagnosed with is chronic fatigue syndrome, a name doctors seem to hand out to any patient with 'unexplained' fatigue, but it is a very real condition. This can be another sign of hypothyroidism not being optimally treated, and once your blood results (a full thyroid panel) read optimally, and you have optimal iron, ferritin, B12 and Vitamin D, etc. it may well just go away or improve a lot. I personally believe that hypothyroidism and adrenal issues are likely behind a lot of chronic fatigue syndrome diagnoses.

## Weight Gain and Exercise Struggles

Since low thyroid levels can lead to weight gain, this can result in being overweight and/or obese.

The main purpose of thyroid hormones, produced by the thyroid gland, is to ensure the metabolism is running properly. And the metabolism's job is to produce heat and fuel. Heat to keep us warm and fuel to give us energy. Now, if we don't have enough of thyroid hormone, our metabolism won't work properly and so can't provide us with adequate heat and fuel.

Therefore, people with an underactive thyroid or hypothyroidism have a slow metabolism, so will have symptoms associated with a slow metabolism, such as cold intolerance (from the lack of heat made) and extreme tiredness and weight gain (from the lack of calories burned to make energy).

Medical professionals seem to think that the weight gain from hypothyroidism is usually between 10 and 30 pounds, thinking that the body adjusts for the slower metabolism after a while. This is very much disputed, though, as many patients carry on gaining, despite a low calorie diet or excessive exercise.

So shouldn't the weight gain stop or come off once you start medication?

Ideally, yes, but not always. It can be more complicated than that. Many patients don't start to see weight loss until their thyroid hormone levels are optimal, as are vitamin levels, have good gut health, adrenal health and concentrate on how they feel physically first. Often natural weight loss occurs once the body is in a healthier place.

Extreme dieting or exercise in a bid to lose weight with hypothyroidism can actually make you *more* hypothyroid and more unwell.

What many thyroid patients don't know is that chronic dieting can reduce Free T3 levels, the active thyroid hormone, causing the metabolism to slow down even further and weight loss to become even more difficult as time goes on. As well as hypothyroidism symptoms to increase or worsen. Studies have even found that dieting can reduce metabolic function and T3 levels. One particular study[36] showed that even seven days of restricting calories can result in a significant reduction of T3. It resulted in a 25% reduction in T3, which, as already explained, can affect everything including your energy levels and metabolic function. In conclusion, during caloric restriction, transport of T4 and T3 into tissues was diminished.

When it comes to exercise, repeatedly engaging in overly demanding exercise can cause a surge of biochemical imbalances to occur within the body, including the disruption of the hypothalamus-pituitary axis, which can reduce thyroid function. Intense cardio, marathon running and training, obsessive weight lifting etc. with little to no recovery time can all cause extreme stress to the body and particularly thyroid health. When the body is under stress, we know by now that it responds by producing cortisol, a stress hormone produced by the adrenal glands. Many of us with hypothyroidism already have stressed-out and overworked adrenal glands, due to the stress of having hypothyroidism, even without knowing. This means that we could have high cortisol levels already, where our body is in a constant stressed-out mode, and producing more cortisol by overexerting ourselves only makes this worse.

When cortisol is overly produced, it can inhibit thyroid function and cause adrenal dysfunction, where, even if our thyroid test results look OK, we still feel rubbish.

You may think you are following a perfectly healthy workout routine, when in reality you could actually be causing some serious damage to your body. It is important for us to know therefore when enough is enough and when we need to slow things down. Listening to our bodies is crucial and taking things at our own pace will help us avoid causing any issues with over exercising.

Although there *are* benefits to higher intensity training, such as burning more body fat and building lean muscle, without maintaining a good balance of exercising, resting and recuperating, along with proper nutrition, setbacks in our health and symptoms can plague us.

Physical activities that tend to be popular among thyroid patients include: yoga, Pilates, swimming, walking and even dancing. Anything that can be done in the comfort of your own home and at your own pace is a big plus and if you can add a social aspect into it too – perhaps getting friends to support you – even better! Avoid any exercise that is clearly hindering you, worsening your health, makes any of your thyroid symptoms worse, or is too intensive or high-impact. As well as the type of exercise, consider how often your body is happy to do it, too.

It may not benefit from a 5k run every day, but a 45-minute walk can work really well instead. You may need to apply some trial and error as you give a few different types of exercise a go and see how your body reacts. You want to be promoting more energy instead of only draining yourself further. You should feel energised and happy after exercise, not worse off! Always increase intensity and frequency slowly and if your body struggles, listen to it.

When it comes to weight gain and weight fluctuations with hypothyroidism, I do understand the frustrations. My weight has fluctuated quite a lot with hypothyroidism and what I've learnt in my bid to try and lose weight with frequent yo-yo dieting and calorie restrictions, is that my physical health is so much more important than how I look in the mirror, or my weight alone. Often, if we focus on feeling physically well, our bodies shed any extra pounds that it doesn't need anyway.

I just want thyroid patients to be aware that often, dieting and calorie restrictions place extra stress upon the body, that it just doesn't need when it's already battling chronic illnesses and hormone imbalances such as hypothyroidism. And we can feel worse because of them, hindering our own recovery.

As well as the studies that demonstrate how dieting can in fact make you more hypothyroid, the effects of denying yourself adequate fuel in the form of food, can include fatigue, drowsiness, blood sugar imbalances, mental health risks and more, in terms of physical proof. You're not likely to recover from your health conditions if you're denying it adequate nutrition, fuel, rest and exercise that *agrees* with your body.

**Alzheimer's Disease**

Particularly interesting and quite scary, is Alzheimer's Disease being connected to your thyroid levels. A study[37] found that:

*"Women with TSH below 1.0 and those with a TSH above 2.1 had a greater than two-fold higher risk of developing Alzheimer's Disease."*

In contrast, they observed no such relationship between TSH levels and Alzheimer's Disease risk in men.

## Chapter Recap:

- Treating and managing your thyroid condition is like piecing back together a big jigsaw puzzle. There can be different pieces for different people, but it is important to find out what yours are and address them.

- As well as other conditions existing alongside hypothyroidism, some conditions can even be caused by low thyroid hormone levels. Even when you're on medication.

- The importance of optimal levels can't be stressed enough for correcting other issues.

# Chapter 5: Thyroid Flare Ups

*"It's OK to have non-perfect health days." - Rachel Hill, The Invisible Hypothyroidism*

*Body weighed down, hot and cold flushes, room spinning, migraine, legs like jelly.* That's what a thyroid flare up often looks like for me. I wake up in the morning knowing I am in a flare, feeling more tired than when I went to bed the night before and my body feels as if it is being weighed down. I struggle to move around and feel dazed. I struggle to work on flare days, but I've sure tried to in the past.

I'll put on some basic makeup – mascara and lip balm – and run a brush through my hair before pushing it back in to a ponytail. I sit at my desk and attempt to work but my head pounds, the room spins, I can't sit up straight and my body flashes with scorching heat. After telling myself I can push on through for so long, I eventually call it quits, close the laptop and tears burst out of my eyes. I stand up from the desk chair but my legs buckle.

This is the reality of someone with hypothyroidism and Hashimoto's on a bad day. Flare ups can really catch me off guard but they've become something I must accept and not beat myself up for. When they come, I feel like I'm in somebody else's body. I've had thyroid flare days when my hypothyroidism hasn't been under control *and* when it has. You may not have even realised that thyroid flare ups were a thing, but they totally are!

## What Is a 'Thyroid Flare Up'?

A Hashimoto's or thyroid flare is defined by an increase in symptoms of the condition/s. A flare usually occurs for a few days to a few weeks.

Symptoms can differ from person to person, though the most commonly reported in a flare up are:

- Increased fatigue
- Heaviness (as if your body is being weighed down)
- Worsened mental health
- Brain fog
- Migraines
- Flu-like symptoms (aches and pains)
- Switching between feeling really cold and really hot

## What Causes a Flare Up?

These are my most common triggers, along with many other thyroid patients I've spoken to over the years:

- Drinking alcohol
- Eating poorly (such as a lot of sugary or processed food, not giving your body good nutrition)
- Consuming a known food allergen or sensitivity (such as gluten, dairy, soy etc.)
- Overexertion (mentally and/or physically) – See the spoons post

- Stress
- Not sticking to a good sleep routine
- Viral, bacterial, fungal etc. infections
- Being on your period or due to start on your period, pregnancy (hormonal fluctuations)

Each time you experience a flare up, try to pinpoint what things (such as those listed above) could have contributed to it. The main thing to do then is avoid those triggers in future (where you can), so as to reduce the chances of another flare.

Some people also find relief from flare-ups when they eliminate a food allergy or sensitivity, such as gluten or dairy. You can also look at quieting the immune response by lowing your thyroid antibodies if you have Hashimoto's. By lowering thyroid antibodies, we're told that this puts the condition under control and means it is better managed. Much of this book contains the things you can do to lower thyroid antibodies and you'll find what specifically lowered mine in Chapter 2.

Supporting your immune system and body as a whole with good nutrition, supplements such as Vitamin C, D and Selenium, adequate sleep and keeping stress levels low can all help.

Ensuring you are addressing any adrenal dysfunction is also very key, as adrenal fatigue (though it is more accurately referred to as hypothalamic-pituitary axis dysfunction) often goes hand in hand with hypothyroidism and can cause many of the same symptoms. Having your thyroid levels tested regularly and ensuring they're all optimised is very important.

131

Learning how to implement and maintain good balance in all aspects of your life is crucial, so make sure you use the spoon theory to work on this.

## How To Manage Flare Ups When They Happen

First and foremost, it is important to say that if you're feeling incredibly unwell, then you should always see your doctor in case something more serious is going on.

The bad thyroid days are a part of having hypothyroidism that I have learnt to accept with time, but I did, at one point, think I would be able to make a 100% recovery, meaning that I would never have any bad thyroid health days ever again. But you know what? No *one* person is in perfect health every single day of their lives. And so, it's perfectly normal to expect flare ups in symptoms from time to time. Don't beat yourself up about this. My (and your) health is always going to require close monitoring to try and keep it on track as much as possible.

On a bad thyroid day or flare up day, it can help to keep yourself warm, rested, well hydrated and well fed. You can put on some films or your favourite TV show to take your mind off the unpleasant symptoms, drink lots of warm drinks such as hot water and lemon or herbal teas, eat nourishing food, enjoy bone broths and even call a friend or two for support. But if you don't feel sociable, then that's OK too. Listen to your body and let it have whatever it needs in order to get over this flare. The sooner you recover, the better for you.

On days where I have to work or otherwise don't have the luxury of just resting in front of the TV or in bed, I'll compromise. I can try to limit how much work or other commitments impede my recovery from a flare up. For example, seeking permission to work from home, working altered hours until the flare has passed, replacing walking to and from work with transport to save energy, or otherwise speaking to my line manager about suitable adjustments.

If making changes surrounding my work isn't an option, at the very least I support recuperating outside of work as much as possible. I limit how much unnecessary activity I do and maximise resting and recuperation time instead. Learn to say "no". I avoid sugar and caffeine and other stimulants that place additional stress on the endocrine system, and eat nutrient dense food to nourish me and aid my recovery. If I can, I'll take a bath and relax, listen to music… anything that helps me feel good. But most importantly: I try to take it easy.

Don't over-do anything in a flare up, as this will likely make it worse, so instead listen to your body and do not in any way overexert it during a flare up. Don't do anything requiring too much from you mentally, physically or emotionally.

Flare ups are only temporary, so if you're experiencing tough symptoms regularly, it is likely not just a flare up but something else more long-term that needs addressing. Using the resources in this book (and those listed at the end of the book) will help you to unearth this and make long-term health improvements.

If you follow me on my blog or social media, then you'll see that I often share my thyroid flare up days quite openly and honestly in order to raise more awareness on this aspect of thyroid conditions.

## Chapter Recap:

- Thyroid flare ups are a common part of living with hypothyroidism and Hashimoto's.

- You may be able to trace your flare up back to a trigger, but these are not always obvious.

- There are various things you can try to prevent having as many flare ups in future and these help many people to control their thyroid condition better.

- When in a flare up, prioritise your recuperation in any way you can.

# Chapter 6: You've Got to Nourish to Flourish

*"I don't trust people who don't love food." – Rachel Hill, The Invisible Hypothyroidism*

I am a foodie, through and through. I have always loved food and always will. When we have health conditions, such as a thyroid condition, food and good nutrition can become even more important, however.

I always say that everything we eat has the power to either help or hinder our health, including our thyroid health and how well our thyroid condition is managed. When we're mindful about what we eat and drink and how we fuel our bodies, we are often rewarded with improved energy levels, clearer heads, better gut health and regular bowel movements, as well as healthier skin, hair and nails. I also notice that my mental health is a lot better when I pay attention to what I eat, too. When I eat rubbish, I feel rubbish. It can even lead to a flare up.

A part of advocating for our health and taking control includes being mindful and intentional about what we put into our bodies and understanding how this can affect how we feel, too. Food is yummy, yes, but it is also fuel for our bodies and this can either be good or bad fuel.

Now, I'm not one for encouraging diets that limit foods and due to my past history of disordered eating/eating disorders, I encourage people to focus on eating healthily and what helps them to feel good. So, don't think I'm about to tell you one hundred things that you shouldn't be eating.

This chapter will hopefully help you to decide what changes to make to your nutrition, in order to help yourself.

## Food Sensitivities

The most common food sensitivities in those with hypothyroidism include gluten, dairy, soy, nightshades and other grains. However, you may not show signs of sensitivity to any of these, or you may be sensitive to *all* of them. You may need to avoid some other foods, too. It really is all individual.

I have been gluten-free for years now, as it has resolved many of my thyroid symptoms, but when I was dairy-free for several months, it did nothing for me whatsoever. So, finding out what works for you is really important.

The most common way of finding out which foods affect us, is via the Elimination Provocation Diet (EPD). The idea of the EPD is to initially remove all and any foods which may be making your thyroid health worse, before adding them back in one by one and looking for noticeable responses to these foods.

Those wanting to try the EPD are generally advised to remove all potentially inflammatory foods from their diet for three weeks.

These include:

- Gluten
- Dairy

- Corn

- Eggs

- Nightshades

- Nuts

- Legumes

- Shellfish

- Citrus

- Soy

After three weeks, the reintroduction of each food type can slowly begin. On a 'reintroduction day' you would choose one food type to reintroduce back in to your diet, eating around five servings in one day whilst monitoring symptoms over the next few days to determine if it needs to stay out of your diet for good. Keeping a food diary can be incredibly helpful here. Symptoms of a food sensitivity may include fatigue, heartburn, indigestion, bloating, gas, muscle aches and pains, joint pain, skin issues, brain fog etc. but can be individual to you. If it causes any undesirable symptoms, it's probably best removed for good.

The foods from the list can then continue to be reintroduced into your diet one at a time, every few days, and signs of issues with these foods recorded.

As well as finding out which foods are making your health worse and removing these from your diet for good, it's helpful to be aware of what other foods you should be eating in abundance and which you should be avoiding for optimal thyroid health.

Others to avoid can include soy, which is a goitrogen that blocks the activity of the TPO enzyme, which has therefore been linked to the development of autoimmune thyroiditis and hypothyroidism. A lot of thyroid patients therefore choose to avoid it. For obvious reasons, sugar and processed foods should also be avoided or limited in everybody, not just thyroid patients. They drive inflammation and disease, something we should be wary of when we have thyroid disease, and can make symptoms worse. They can also contribute to poor gut health (which is incredibly important to our overall health) and encourage blood sugar imbalances. It's best to go back to basics with a lot of food. Get five servings of fruit and five servings of vegetables a day (minimum), and eat with a focus on healthy fats and proteins.

When it comes to goitrogenic foods, the general consensus is to eat them in moderation and that it seems they're only goitrogenic in their raw state. Therefore, many suggest that cooking them adequately removes the goitrogens, or at least a large majority of them. For example, cooking goitrogenic vegetables like broccoli and sprouts until the 'crunch' has gone, can indicate that the goitrogens have also gone. Whilst consuming fermented and cooked cruciferous vegetables is preferred, occasionally eating small amounts of them raw should not aggravate thyroid conditions. The key is moderation really. I don't actively avoid any goitrogenic foods but also do not eat large quantities of them daily.

As someone who has gone gluten-free and seen a lot of benefits, and as a gluten-free diet is the most cited with a thyroid condition, I focus mainly on this diet change when talking about my own experiences. We covered the reasons why many of us react to gluten in Chapters 2 and 4, but how do you go gluten-free?

## How To Go Gluten-Free

On a gluten-free diet, you should avoid any foods that contain:

- Gluten
- Wheat
- Oats (unless they're gluten-free oats)
- Barley
- Rye
- Spelt
- and malt.

You'll probably be surprised at just how much food contains these things, such as some chocolate bars, alcohol, sauces, vinegar and condiments. The obvious foods that contain them also are bread, pasta, pizza, biscuits, cake and porridge. It's often easier to avoid gluten if you avoid processed foods.

It's good to know that most foods are available in gluten-free alternatives and the quality of these are getting better. I have been able to find gluten-free versions of pretty much everything. However, a lot of gluten-free products (such as cake, bread and biscuits) contain a lot of sugar and can be really unhealthy for you and your endocrine health. They're also typically more expensive. Due to the lack of desired taste, texture or look in gluten-free products, companies often fill them with sugar and other not-so-good things to compensate, so you should limit your consumption of gluten-free labelled products to just special occasions.

For example, gluten-free cake, sausage rolls, pizza bases and pasta can be significantly sugarier than their gluten-filled counterparts. You're better using naturally gluten-free alternatives where you can, such as rice noodles in place of regular wheat noodles.

One thing I have discovered and find incredibly interesting, is that better quality and more expensive products tend to be naturally gluten-free. In my local supermarket, the own brand chilled sausages contain wheat (gluten), but the more expensive, 'butcher's selection' ones do not. Another is gravy. With the leading brand of UK gravy granules, their regular granules contain gluten, but their slightly more upmarket version does not. If you think about what that's saying about wheat as an ingredient, it gives you a lot to think about...

You'll need to adopt a strict behaviour of checking every single thing you eat and drink (although drinks are typically less likely to contain gluten). Every ingredients label, everything you eat at a restaurant or family member's house needs to be inspected, so you'll need to really advocate for yourself. If any meal, food or drink you are presented with contains gluten (in the forms listed above) you cannot eat it.

As time goes on, you'll recognise the typical culprits that contain gluten, so eating out and around a friend's house will become easier. For example, I tend to order meat, vegetables and salad dishes when out as they are naturally free from gluten (and are generally healthy too), but you can ask the restaurant for their gluten-free menu or they will point out the gluten-free options on the regular menu. Just be sure to ask about contamination issues i.e. how food is prepared.

Cross-contamination means that gluten-free meals have been prepared on surfaces and in the same pots as gluten-containing food, e.g. chips/fries that are naturally gluten free, being fried in the same oil as onion rings (gluten alert!) which contaminates them. Cooks may also be using the same surface to prepare regular burgers and gluten-free burgers. Generally, I ask when I order food if it is prepared separately to gluten-containing foods, and if it is cooked/fried separately to anything else altogether e.g. no shared oil or equipment. On a gluten-free diet, it's important not to eat any foods cross-contaminated with other gluten-containing food, as it undoes all your hard work.

The easiest way to control cross-contamination is by eating and preparing as much food at home as you can. You'll need to bear in mind that if you live with someone else who eats gluten, then separate cooking equipment will be needed, e.g. separate toasters for bread and separate utensils such as wooden spoons, which can hold on to gluten, will be needed.

In my house, my husband and I have our own toasters, and we mark the wooden spoons, to show which have been used in gluten-containing foods and which are safe and free of gluten.

You may find that take away food is probably the hardest when it comes to gluten-free options. Many do not offer their allergen information online, so you may need to call the restaurant directly and ask them to make sure there is no gluten in the items you're ordering. You will also need to check that they are prepared and cooked separately to avoid cross-contamination. If you don't trust them or they sound unsure, don't risk it. It's not worth feeling ill!

The take away cuisines I tend to avoid are Italian/pizza, Chinese, Korean etc. as they really don't usually have much I can eat, if anything at all. However, Indian, Caribbean, Vietnamese, French etc. are much easier. Thai and Mexican can be mixed.

When it comes to oats, pure oatmeal (oats) are naturally gluten-free, however, many oats are contaminated due to being processed in facilities that also process wheat, barley, and rye (which contain gluten). Any oats that you eat, including those used in products such as flapjacks, must be labelled gluten-free or free from contamination to be safe for you to eat.

When it comes to alcohol, cider, wine, sherry, spirits, port and liqueurs tend to be gluten-free, but do check the specific brand you're drinking. With alcohol, some people following a gluten-free diet can get confused because gluten containing cereals are often used in making alcohol, but the gluten is removed when it is distilled. All spirits are distilled; therefore, this process removes any trace of gluten from the drink. So, all spirit drinks (including malt whisky which is made from barley) are safe for gluten-free people to consume.

Alcohol to definitely avoid includes beer, lager, stout and ale, which contain varying amounts of gluten and are not suitable for a gluten-free diet, but also any spirits or other alcoholic drinks that are flavoured using things like malt. Specially manufactured gluten-free beers, lagers and ales are available in many shops now.

Gluten can appear in some medicine and supplements, so ensure you're not taking in any gluten from those sources either. Talk to your doctor or pharmacist about alternatives if you are.

When it comes to beauty products, look out for:

- Hydrolyzed wheat gluten
- Triticum vulgare (wheat) gluten
- Avena sativa (oat) kernel flour
- Hydrolyzed oat flour
- Secale cereale (rye) seed flour
- Barley extract
- Fermented grain extract
- Hydrolyzed malt extract
- Phytosphingosine extract
- Wheat germ
- Hydrolyzed wheat protein
- Hydrolyzed vegetable protein
- Triticum aestivum (another name for wheat)

What we put on our skin is absorbed, at least to some extent, in to our bodies. Many don't realise that they can be glutening themselves through shampoo or body lotions.

If you're feeling clued up on how to change to a gluten-free diet and feel ready to go, but want to *slowly* integrate going gluten-free in to your life, this isn't really beneficial. Eating any amount of gluten, whether once a week or all day every day, is doing damage to you internally if you have a sensitivity or intolerance. So, eating even a small amount is still harmful. I've been told numerous times that gluten hangs around in the body for up to six months! And every time you eat it, if you have Hashimoto's, it triggers an attack on your thyroid, causing more thyroid tissue to be destroyed and so more thyroid function lost. So, you're best to go gluten-free completely at the start of the week and stick with it. People generally start to see improvements in their health within a few months, though I noticed it by week three.

If you go gluten-free, feel the benefits and decide to keep it up, but occasionally get 'glutened', here are some tips for overcoming the glutening as swiftly as possible:

## Don't Beat Yourself up About It

Whether someone else has glutened you, despite you quizzing them on ingredients, or whether you've accidentally glutened yourself, being hard on yourself afterwards isn't going to help. What you need to do now is focus on getting your body over it as soon as possible.

## Drink Plenty of Water

Doing so helps to flush the gluten through your system quicker and keeps you hydrated if you're having unpleasant toilet trips from being glutened. If ingesting gluten causes you constipation, bloating or wind, you can also try hot drinks such as half a lemon freshly squeezed in to some water, or herbal tea, as these can help to move things along. Lemons also contain antioxidant compounds that activate detoxifying enzymes.

## Eat Chia Seeds

Chia seeds are also great for getting your bowels moving, so you can add these simple seeds to your food for the next few days to help your body expel the gluten. They're also quite high in anti-inflammatory omega-3 fatty acids, which help to reduce the inflammation caused by ingesting gluten.

## Incorporate Turmeric and Ginger

Turmeric and ginger are great natural and inexpensive anti-inflammatories. Ginger can even help to ease stomach cramping.

## Get Bone Broth Down You

Drinking Bone broth is helpful as it is high in anti-inflammatories and amino acids and helps to protect and heal the mucosal lining of the digestive tract that can get disrupted by being glutened.

## Take Probiotics

Probiotics are helpful when taken daily anyway, as they help our guts and support the immune system. You may want to increase your probiotic intake for a few days after gluten ingestion.

## Get Digesting

Digestive enzymes help to speed up the breakdown and absorption of macronutrients, so you can take an enzyme to help move things along. Dipeptidyl peptidase (DPP-IV) can help to break down gluten specifically.

## Rest and Recuperate

If being glutened has caused heavy fatigue, inflammation leading to painful joints, achy muscles or even brain fog, remember to listen to your body and rest if you need it. Being glutened can cause your thyroid condition to flare up. We often push ourselves more than is ideal and can cause a setback in our health. So, listen to your body.

## Alcohol

Alcohol can also be problematic for many thyroid patients. Many of us seem to notice that we feel the effects of alcohol more, since being hypothyroid.

This could be due to your thyroid health and liver health working together, as we know that alcohol can be a stress on the liver (where a lot of thyroid hormone conversion takes place), which processes and metabolises the alcohol you consume. Alcohol is actually known to have a direct toxic effect on thyroid cells, which is used therapeutically in ethanol ablation therapy of thyroid nodules.

Regularly drinking a lot of alcohol also inhibits thyroid hormones T3 and T4 and may reduce the activity of type II 5'-deiodinase. This enzyme is used to convert storage hormone T4 into active hormone T3, and if it is not functioning optimally, you may experience reduced levels of Free T3 with ongoing symptoms. It has also been found that excess alcohol intake blocks the release of TSH.

Alcohol is also oestrogenic, which causes the level of oestrogen in your body to rise, and oestrogen is known to suppress or block thyroid function and hormones from working as efficiently as they should be. This can make you feel extra hypothyroid or even intolerant of alcohol. It can encourage break-outs in some women, especially if they already have oestrogen dominance, along with PMS and delayed periods. It certainly does in me.

Therefore, alcohol can also encourage or contribute to oestrogen dominance, which is a big thyroid jigsaw puzzle piece for many of us.

In response to rising oestrogen, the body can become stressed and on high alert, releasing stress hormones such as cortisol. This can further inhibit the liver from converting T4 to T3 which again, can contribute to us feeling unwell with increased likeliness of adrenal dysfunction. Increased cortisol can deplete progesterone levels further, resulting in even higher oestrogen levels, feeding back in to oestrogen dominance. It can be a vicious cycle!

Alcohol can also deplete minerals and vitamins such as magnesium, folic acid, B Vitamins and Selenium, all of which are very important for thyroid health and many of us have low levels in these or struggle to absorb them due to impaired gut health.

As a result of all of this, when you consume alcohol and also have hypothyroidism, you may feel extra hypothyroid the next day or even take several days to recover from it, feeling extra tired and achy. Thyroid flare ups can occur as a result of alcohol when you have hypothyroidism. However, not all thyroid patients report alcohol making them feel this way, so as with everything, it's all individual. Personally, I stopped drinking alcohol a while ago as it just didn't seem to be worth the flare ups that ensued. If alcohol contributes to *you* feeling worse, particularly in the form of a flare up of thyroid symptoms, consider whether it is best to avoid it to better manage your health. Everyone should be mindful of their alcohol consumption anyway and make sure to limit it to just a few drinks a week ideally.

## Caffeine

I know a lot of you won't like me adding caffeine to this list, but it is worth being aware of how it can make endocrine health issues worse.

Caffeine increases our blood sugar levels when consumed. Blood sugar spikes cause cortisol to shoot up, which can tire out the adrenals and exacerbate hypoglycaemia, Hashimoto's and 'adrenal fatigue'. When your blood sugar levels drop below normal, sometimes after a spike, your adrenal glands respond by secreting more cortisol. This cortisol then tells the liver to produce more glucose, which brings blood sugar levels back to normal. Doing this repeatedly can cause abnormal cortisol output and can suppress pituitary function.

Drinking coffee whilst also having 'adrenal fatigue' adds fuel to the fire and can make it worse, so it is often best avoided whilst adrenal issues are present. However, many thyroid patients are able to go back to drinking it once this is resolved.

Coffee can also irritate the oesophagus or weaken the lower oesophageal sphincter, which prevents the backward flow of stomach contents that causes acid reflux. Coffee is highly acidic, so it stimulates the release of gastrin and bile. For people with autoimmune conditions and compromised digestion, this can cause further digestive damage to the intestinal lining.

Caffeine can trigger migraines and headaches, which many of us with hypothyroidism also seem to experience. Since caffeine narrows the blood vessels that surround your brain, when you don't consume it, they expand again, and this can cause pain. It's easy for your body to get used to caffeine, and when you don't have it in your system, you can have a withdrawal headache or migraine. As explained previously, the spike in blood sugar caused by caffeine could also cause headaches.

Some women experience migraines around the time of their period, possibly because of changes in the level of oestrogen and progesterone, so it's worth knowing that caffeine affects oestrogen levels too. Studies have shown that women who consumed at least 500mg of caffeine daily, the equivalent of four or five cups of coffee, had nearly 70% more oestrogen than women who consumed no more than 100mg of caffeine daily (less than one cup of coffee). Tea is not much better as it contains about half the amount of caffeine compared to coffee. Migraines, heavy periods, PMT, lumpy breasts and cellulite can be signs of oestrogen dominance.

Coffee contributes to oestrogen dominance, which can inhibit T4 to T3 conversion. Conversion issues with thyroid medication seem very common and can be the reason why your medication doesn't seem to be helping.

However, coffee is not something that usually needs to be avoided for life by most of us with hypothyroidism. Many of us can enjoy it in reasonable amounts, though may benefit from avoiding it whilst overcoming adrenal issues or oestrogen dominance, and reintroducing it after these are addressed.

## Good Foods for Hypothyroidism

The omega-3 fatty acids found in fish such as wild salmon, trout, tuna, or sardines make fish an excellent part of any hypothyroid patient's diet. Hypothyroidism can increase the risk for heart disease as a result of higher levels of LDL, the 'bad' type of cholesterol, so fish rich in omega 3 can lower the risk for heart disease. Fish can also be a source of selenium, which is most concentrated in the thyroid and needed for good thyroid health.

Like Omega-3, other healthy fats such as olive oil, that found in avocados, butter and coconut oil help to keep cholesterol at healthy levels, in order to produce the hormones our bodies need.

Brazil nuts can be high in selenium (if you're able to confirm the nutritional value and content) and can help you to get a good amount for optimal thyroid health, making them a good snack and balancer of blood sugar.

Beans are a good protein source, so are great for sustained energy, which, when you live with hypothyroidism, you may be lacking. They're also high in fibre, which can be helpful if you suffer with constipation, a common side effect of hypothyroidism. You can use them in stews, curries or even salads.

Constipation is a common symptom of hypothyroidism and foods rich in fibre can help this. They can also help balance out wobbly blood sugar which is often coupled with hypothyroidism and help you feel fuller. Just make sure to avoid eating loads of fibre-rich foods near to taking your thyroid medication, as this can affect absorption.

Bone broth encourages a healthy gut which in turn helps with nutrient absorption, Many people with hypothyroidism will also find themselves low in vitamins such as D, B12 or iron. Bone broth can also help with joint pain and gives the immune system a boost as it is full of so much goodness.

Seaweed and kelp are high in iodine and without enough the thyroid gland can swell, also causing the amount of thyroid hormone in your body to drop. They provide other trace minerals too, including iron, calcium, and potassium. It is possible to consume too much iodine, so enjoy in moderation.

When hypothyroidism is autoimmune, you should also consider addressing gut health. A good supply of healthy gut bacteria via fermented foods supports overall good health and for me, improving my gut health was a huge part of improving my thyroid health. Fermented foods such as yogurt and kefir help to continuously stock your gut with beneficial bacteria, resulting in a stronger immune system and overall better health.

Cinnamon, ginger, garlic, peppermint, chamomile and turmeric are anti inflammatories, which can help to control your thyroid condition and promote better health. Many add these to food or take in supplemental/tablet form.

## Chapter Recap:

- Diet changes for improved health can differ from person to person, but knowing how to find out which ones may help you, can be really empowering.

- A gluten-free diet is the most common with hypothyroidism.

- You may benefit from limiting or removing caffeine and alcohol.

- Focusing on eating healthy and fuelling your body with good nutrition can really support your thyroid health as well as energy levels, clear thinking, bowel movements and other thyroid symptoms.

# Chapter 7: My Experience with Medical Professionals

*"Not until we are lost, do we begin to find ourselves."* - *Henry David Thoreau*

Five months into diagnosis and on Levothyroxine, I was still feeling unwell. In fact, I was just feeling worse as the weeks went on. With a growing list of symptoms and complaints, I was really frustrated at my life falling apart - work life, home management, social and personal life. I didn't understand how my levels could always come back 'normal' when I felt so unwell, but as research led me to question the tests my doctor was doing, the medication I was given and told it would 'make me better', I realised I had been lied to. And massively let down.

As I explained in Chapter 3, I eventually made the switch to NDT and, as soon as I started it, I booked an appointment to speak to my regular GP in a weeks' time to discuss it. (Note: I *always* recommend informing your doctor[38]).

The GP I was seeing at this appointment, I hadn't seen before. I decided this was going to be my last attempt at getting NDT prescribed, or else I'd carry on taking the NDT I'd successfully managed to self-source online.

The GP listened, nodded and let me finish everything I wanted to say - read from a letter I'd typed up previously[39], to make sure I'd got everything across that I wanted to. He then calmly began his response to me, with my other half sat in the room for support.

The GP was pleased that I'd already made improvements since beginning the NDT just a few weeks earlier and didn't think it was a coincidence. He admitted that he knew nothing about Natural Desiccated Thyroid medication and so could not prescribe it or dose it for me, but said that he would refer me to an endocrinologist as they may be able to.

I was over the moon. I had hope that I may be able to get the medication that I needed prescribed. And in that month or so between the appointment with the new GP and my first appointment with the endocrinologist, I was so full of hope.

But this was soon brought down when I had my first appointment with the endocrinologist.

I took him the same letter I read to my GP, and he read it before doing anything else. Afterwards, he lectured me on the risks of using NDT and explained why he would not prescribe it for me. He said it hadn't proven to be any better than Levothyroxine, and when I explained it had been, he just needed to open his eyes to the books, research, studies and large body of patients out there, he had no answer.

As expected, he was praising Levothyroxine and trying to convince me of its high success rate. I explained I had been in touch with a large number of thyroid patients online, and it certainly was not as successful as he thought it was. He refused to really listen to anything I had to say about my independent research, as of course, I'm just a patient. What do I know? I only live with this condition, after all.

He then proceeded to ask me about my symptoms and how I felt NDT had helped me more so than Levothyroxine. I explained how, on Levothyroxine, I had over twenty symptoms and that while only being on NDT for a month so far, all but one symptom had gone. He put it down to coincidence, and said that, given enough time on Levothyroxine, I would have had the same experience. However, I was on Levothyroxine for six months and got nothing but worse, whilst doctors insisted that my TSH was 'fine', therefore I was 'fine' and all these symptoms were in my head. So I didn't believe this at all.

Anyway, we eventually moved past that and I explained how the one symptom left was my fatigue. Still constantly tired, and when I say tired, I don't mean 'you had a late night and are a bit groggy today' tired, I mean absolutely exhausted.

When I explained my level of fatigue and the poor stamina that came along with it, the endocrinologist decided to diagnose me with chronic fatigue syndrome, and said that it would get better 'over time'. His favourite phrase was *"these things are often only 'time-limited.'"* When I asked why, he couldn't give me an answer. I felt it was a total cop-out, a lame excuse for saying he didn't know, and he didn't really care enough about me, his patient, to explore it further.

I suggested it could be caused by adrenal dysfunction, since my last set of blood results came back with a TSH in range, Free T4 in range and Free T3 over the range. Adrenal issues (such as high cortisol) can cause T3 to 'pool' in your blood, making the result look really high. And here comes my favourite part. He looked at me and said, *"just by looking at you, I can tell you do not have adrenal issues."*

And I was gobsmacked.

Just by looking at me last year, you wouldn't have been able to tell that I was hypothyroid, yet I know it was really starting to cause me problems back then. It was in full swing! I *was* ill and just by looking at me, no one believed me. I was an active and busy, healthy looking twenty-year-old, yet my bodily processes were shutting down one by one and I was constantly fighting against it controlling me and my life. This is a common problem we thyroid patients have. We often don't look 'ill enough' to be taken seriously, and it needs to change.

I left the appointment, cried a lot in frustration, and then ordered my own adrenal stress test to be done privately. This was the first of many tests I ordered myself and it was easy peasy, as well as very empowering. Within two weeks I had my results which showed that my adrenal glands were indeed dysfunctioning. My cortisol output was elevated significantly in the morning and up to lunch time, and although 'in range' in the afternoon and evening, it was still at the top of the 'acceptable range'. My cortisol was too high 24/7. Abnormal adrenal results!

And so, my first endocrinologist appointment was basically a waste of time, but at least I had the opportunity which is a lot more than what many other thyroid patients seem to get. However, from what I hear from other thyroid patients in my support group about their visits to endocrinologists, they're generally not much more fruitful than mine. Not all, I must stress, but a lot.

For another year and a half, I carried on managing my thyroid health mostly by myself, visiting my NHS GP for a thyroid panel testing of TSH, Free T3 and Free T4 (he was happy to do this every few months) and tweaking my NDT dose as it seemed fit, with his input too. For most of the time, my levels were optimal and I gradually felt more and more well as time went on, but every now and then they would demonstrate adrenal stress with a Free T3 suddenly shooting above range and 'pooling'. I knew my adrenal dysfunction wasn't improving and following another self-ordered test six months after the original, it showed that they had only gotten worse.

So, I eventually took the plunge in searching for a functional medicine practitioner - a private doctor or healthcare practitioner who practises the functional medicine approach. Functional medicine is hugely popular with thyroid patients but I felt daunted by the associated costs for so long.

I soon found a functional medicine practitioner who would work within my budget, and, in just a few months, I was making huge progress on my leaky gut, candida, sex hormone imbalance and adrenal fatigue. The final pieces of my thyroid jigsaw puzzle came together and my life was healthy, happy and not ruled by my thyroid anymore.

You see, in a day and age where doctors are now more pushed for time than ever, limited in terms of budgets and are overworked, many thyroid patients don't get the treatment they need to feel better. Especially with mainstream medicine. Public health systems do not necessarily allocate funding to allow doctors to get patients the right treatments and tests required. They often dismiss people wanting to play an active role in their own healthcare. Doctors rarely have the time to listen to us in enough detail.

## Types of Medical Practitioners Who Can Treat Hypothyroidism

The majority of this book is based on functional medicine practises and as such, you may well find that your conventional medicine endocrinologist or doctor dismisses a lot of what is shared here, as well as among other thyroid advocates. But that isn't to say it's not true. This is where being your own health advocate is crucial, as like me, you may struggle to get your conventional medicine doctor to look in to or try some of the things mentioned in this book.

As a thyroid patient newly embracing being my own thyroid advocate, it was frustrating to time and time again, read about a new thing I wanted to try or a test I wanted doing and coming up against a conventional medicine practitioner who laughed it off and denied that it had any relevance. This is particularly common in the UK.

So, ordering your own tests, doing your own trials and research and even seeking out the help of an alternative medical practitioner such as a naturopath or functional doctor may be beneficial to you. I don't want to tell you all the things that have gotten me better in this book, only for you to go to your GP and have them turn you away disappointedly. I soon learnt to be prepared for this reaction from my GP but that was OK, because I was getting better at advocating for myself and finding other ways to get those tests done or try a new intervention.

As a thyroid patient, there are a few different types of doctors or medical professionals you may see for your condition. Some can be more useful in addressing different areas of the condition than others and different patients find different levels of success with different *types* of medical professionals. You may have tried a few of these already, but I'm going to sum up *what* each one is, *how* they look at hypothyroidism and *why* they may be helpful to you.

First of all, let's begin with an explanation on:

## Conventional Medicine VS Functional Medicine

In Western medicine, there are two main approaches to medicine, conventional and functional, the former being what it says on the tin – conventional ways to treat a patient e.g. they come in with a symptom so they're given a drug to help with that – but functional medicine looks at the root cause of the symptoms, and fixing that, before jumping to treating just the symptoms with drugs.

Endocrinologists and GPs generally fall into conventional medicine, as well as some private doctors. However, I see a private GP who combines conventional and integrative medicine practises. Whereas Conventional medicine looks at each symptom and health condition as a separate issue to treat, functional medicine is holistic and looks at the whole body, considering how one issue can have a knock-on effect and cause other things to go wrong, too.

Whilst also considering *some* drugs, functional medicine places importance on lifestyle factors such as diet – what we eat and drink – stress levels, chemicals, toxins and much more. For some people, conventional medicine does them just fine and they return to good health on thyroid medication alone for their thyroid condition, but for many others, they never *quite* feel right again, post-hypothyroidism diagnosis and conventional doctors prescribe multiple medicines for multiple symptoms that we are told, are *separate* issues.

A lot of thyroid patients therefore feel a functional medicine approach is better suited to them because it not only deals with their thyroid condition, but also looks at other parts of the endocrine system which may have also gone awry, such as those pesky adrenal glands and sex hormones, and it works to bring them back into balance, also addressing any other issues from the root, avoiding the need for a growing list of prescription medications.

Functional practitioners also consider whether your hypothyroidism is autoimmune (it is for around 90% of us) as being very important and crucial in your recovery. Conventional medicine feel that treatment will always remain the same, whether you have autoimmune thyroid disease or not. Due to cost restraints, conventional doctors are rarely able to use innovative tests and treatments and often can't spend enough time to help identify, run tests or treat complex autoimmune diseases and hormonal imbalances. So, when you need more personalised thyroid treatment, conventional medicine can feel inadequate.

## GP

In the UK, and many Western countries, GPs are the most common first port of call. GP stands for general practitioner. They don't tend to be specialists in a particular area or field and as such, tend to know a standard amount about all aspects of the body, rather than being focused on one area or system alone.

GPs are generally the people who diagnose hypothyroidism in most cases and many thyroid patients see their GP for thyroid medication prescriptions, dosage adjustments and any on-going issues. However, they can refer you to a thyroid specialist if you have on-going complaints of symptoms and conventional T4-only medication (Levothyroxine or Synthroid for example) not working as well as you'd hoped. Some thyroid patients do just fine on the standard medication and simple dosage adjustments their GP can make, but for those who are still not feeling optimised for their condition, a referral to an endocrinologist can be made and may be useful. Most commonly, in the UK GPs tend to follow a conventional medicine approach and can only prescribe T4-only medication.

## Endocrinologist

An endocrinologist (often called an *endo* for short) specialises in the endocrine system, a system that includes the thyroid gland as well as the hypothalamus, pituitary, parathyroid, adrenal glands, pineal gland, and the reproductive organs (ovaries and testes). The pancreas is also a part of this system; it has a role in hormone production as well as digestion. The endocrine system is made up of glands that produce and secrete hormones. These hormones regulate the body's growth, metabolism and sexual function and an endocrinologist specialises in knowing all the ins and outs of these systems and hormone balances (or, *imbalances*, as many of us have!).

As mentioned above, a referral to an endocrinologist can be made by your GP, but patients are often waiting for months or even years to finally see one. In the UK, you can see an endocrinologist on the NHS. Endocrinologists are somewhat a controversial topic among thyroid patients and others who live with adrenal and reproductive hormone issues, too. Whereas some patients find a good level of success with an endocrinologist, others feel that they follow conventional medicine too closely and thus, are not much more help than their GP.

Sticking to the 'importance' of the TSH test, although paying a bit more attention to other thyroid tests such as

Free T4 and Free T3, endocrinologist's can offer a bit more of a detailed insight in to your thyroid condition and management, including a few more tests (which, to be honest, we should all be having done anyway) but they generally stick to very stiff, outdated ranges and place the most importance on TSH levels.

Depending on where you are in the world, endocrinologist's *can* offer more than T4-only medication but often only prefer to prescribe conventional T4 synthetics. This means getting them to prescribe you T3 and NDT medications, which help many thyroid patients get their good quality of life back, can be difficult. But it is possible. More so in the US than other countries – it is pretty uncommon in the UK for example. Some thyroid patients feel let down after waiting to see an endocrinologist and realising that they're not much more help than their GP, but they *can* be useful. In my opinion, it's always worth trying to see an endocrinologist at least once, so you can decide for yourself.

## Private GP/Private Doctor

Private doctors or private GPs here in the UK especially, tend to fall mostly into conventional medicine practises but often offer more than mainstream doctors, such as that on the NHS. For example, the NHS only offer the thyroid medication Levothyroxine for the most part, but private doctors or GPs can offer more types of thyroid medications. They are often keen to do more in depth and comprehensive testing (such as the full thyroid panel) too, but all of this can cost a lot out of pocket.

I see a private GP doctor who prescribes me my NDT medication, and he combines both mainstream and integrative medical practises and information, and sees himself as a holistic doctor. He's a fan of many of the resources I've listed at the end of this book, including Stop The Thyroid Madness and Dr. Barry Durrant-Peatfield.

## Functional Doctor or Functional Medicine Practitioner

Functional doctors or functional medicine practitioners tend to do more comprehensive testing than conventional ones, look at changing other aspects of your life including diet, routines for sleeping and stress coping and prefer to treat you by looking at the whole body as a system that needs to work in harmony together, rather than focusing on the thyroid gland alone, as conventional medicine does.

Functional doctors/medicine practitioners generally cost more than conventional and in the UK, they're not covered on the NHS. Seeing a functional doctor qualifies as paying to see a private doctor and costs can be quite high, but there are functional doctors out there offering services for different kinds of budgets. It's always worth having an online search and emailing for quotes on prices.

Many thyroid patients turn to functional doctors or practitioners after years of feeling let down by conventional medicine, and there's loads of info online singing their praises. With an approach that looks at the whole body as opposed to just the thyroid and supporting good overall health, it's a more personalised approach to your specific situation. In my experience, a functional medicine practitioner was the way to go when addressing my health as a whole. They focused on my gut, adrenal and sex hormone health in particular.

## Naturopath

A naturopath applies natural therapies to health conditions, often to compliment what you're receiving from a conventional or functional doctor. It includes natural healing practices such as homeopathy, acupuncture, and herbal medicine. They provide personalised care to each patient, and, similar to a functional doctor, they see the body as a holistic unity of body, mind, and spirit, aiming to address the body as one. Not all naturopaths have medical degrees, so whilst some are Naturopathic Doctors, others are simply Naturopaths. Only those with medical degrees can write prescriptions. Like functional medicine doctors or practitioners, you would usually pay to see a naturopath and costs can range to suit various budgets.

## Obstetrician or Gynaecologist

Obstetricians and gynaecologists can also help to manage thyroid conditions. These obstetrics specialists are generally concerned with the care of a pregnant woman, her unborn child and the management of diseases specific to women, such as thyroid issues, which can come to light during pregnancy, be triggered by pregnancy or get better or worse during pregnancy.

Managing hypothyroidism in pregnancy is of paramount importance to reduce risks of complications and miscarriage. In gynaecology, patients range from those who have chronic disorders which are not life threatening but interfere significantly with quality of life, such as thyroid disease, to those where an acute emergency presentation is the first indication of a gynaecological problem.

Gynaecology is concerned with the well-being and health of the female reproductive organs and the ability to reproduce, which involves a lot of the endocrine system. When one part of this system goes awry, so can others, so sex hormone imbalances and adrenal issues for example are pretty common with thyroid problems. You will usually be referred to an obstetrician when pregnant or a gynaecologist for reproductive system related symptoms or issues – both are included on the NHS in the UK. Many thyroid patients find that they get more comprehensive thyroid testing done compared to an endocrinologist or GP, from an obstetrician or gynaecologist. If you fall pregnant as a thyroid patient, you may be referred to see an obstetrician or gynaecologist to help manage you through pregnancy.

## ENT Specialist

Ears, Nose and Throat specialists can be involved with the management and treatment of thyroid conditions due to the location of the gland being in the neck. Thyroid patients who are referred to an ENT (can be done on the NHS) are often done so due to complications of their thyroid disease such as goitres, nodules, inflammation or enlargement of the thyroid gland. They recognise autoimmune hypothyroidism (Hashimoto's) and how it can affect the thyroid gland in terms of inflammation. ENT specialists may conduct further testing that an endocrinologist and GP cannot, such as:

- More in-depth blood tests of thyroid function
- An ultrasound examination of your neck and thyroid

- A radioactive thyroid scan
- A fine needle aspiration biopsy

They will pick up on any abnormalities such as thyroid cancer and create a treatment plan going forward for any issues they may diagnose or find.

## So, Who Is the Best Doctor or Practitioner to Treat *Your* Thyroid Condition?

I wish I could tell you! I hope I've at least helped to inform you on your options and encouraged you to be your own advocate, helping you figure out which direction to go to find the best practitioner for you and improve your overall health and wellbeing.

In my own experience, I've made more progress in my health in the first few months of seeing a functional medicine practitioner, compared to years on the NHS alone. Seeing a private GP to get my NDT medication prescribed has also been a huge step.

Finding the right practitioner for you can be time-consuming but very much worth the time. Some tips include asking the thyroid patient community for recommendations (such as in online forums and support groups), using the 'Find a Doctor' page on the American Thyroid Association website, using the 'Find a Provider' option on the Institute for Functional Medicine website, the 'Find a Doctor' page on the ThyroidChange website, googling your area (e.g. 'Functional Doctor in London') or if you're in the UK specifically, you can contact Thyroid UK for their list of private practitioners that are often more open to comprehensive testing and treatment for hypothyroidism.

## Chapter Recap:

- Not every thyroid patient does well on standard treatment and care from their standard doctor/s.
- Just know that there are other medical professionals to help if your first option does not work out.
- You should be your own thyroid advocate whilst working with your medical professional/s of choice.
- You may see a range of medical practitioners which make up your healthcare team.

# Chapter 8: Getting the Most out of Your Medical Appointments

*"No one knows your body better than you do." - Rachel Hill, The Invisible Hypothyroidism*

So many thyroid patients struggle to build a good relationship with a doctor. As I've talked about before, it can be tricky to find a doctor who will test thyroid conditions comprehensively (that is, including the full thyroid panel of tests), consider various thyroid medication options and fully listen to our concerns without playing them off as something else or even implying that they're in our head.

It's understandable therefore, that many of us can feel anxious and worried about medical appointments and struggle to come across as assertive when we need to. Remember, to make the most progress in your health, you should be an active participant in your own healthcare and treatment. After all, you are your own thyroid advocate. Embrace this by learning how to get the most out of your medical appointments.

## Plan Ahead

The number one rule I always give thyroid patients going to see their GP, Endocrinologist or other healthcare professional is to write everything they want to discuss down, ahead of the day.

Have an initial brainstorming session of listing all the symptoms you want to bring up, tests you want to ask for and any other queries or questions and then keep it handy for adding anything else that may come to mind, so you don't leave the appointment annoyed that you'd forgotten to ask something very key to your health and concerns.

It may be easier to keep the list on your phone so it's always with you and you can add to it easily. You may also want to leave some space so you can write the answer or any notes in, to avoid forgetting what was said after the appointment.

At the appointment, simply start by telling the medical professional that you have written some things down and ask them to let you finish before giving their input, so you don't get cut off before you've brought everything up you wish to. Refer back to it often throughout the appointment and ensure you're happy that all has been addressed. If it's quite a long list, consider booking a double appointment slot as doctors can be rushed for time and you'll both benefit from having an adequate timeslot to discuss them properly.

It may also help to have some photos ready depicting any particular symptoms or bad days with your health. When my acne was getting progressively worse, I took daily photos to show just how quickly it was developing and these helped my doctor to understand the extent of my issues and worries better.

If I've recently had any blood tests done, I also like to ask the receptionist to print me out a copy ahead of the appointment so that I have them in front of me when the doctor discusses them (and also to keep in my own file back home). Having test results printed can also help you to pick up on anything the doctor may have missed, such as a 'borderline' or low in range results that the doctor would otherwise say is OK, but you can raise in the appointment. Low in range or borderline results are notorious for still leaving thyroid patients feeling unwell. Many feel better when treatment moves their results further in to the reference range.

## Support

Consider whether taking someone else along to your appointment for support will help. After getting fed up with feeling like no one was taking me seriously, I started taking my long-term partner (now-husband) along to appointments and I suddenly started getting places quicker.

Although it definitely shouldn't take someone else backing you up in order to be listened to, many doctors will see it as validation to what you're saying. If you can take someone who lives with you then even better, as they can explain how they see hypothyroidism affect you each and every day.

## Backup

If you're wanting to try another type of thyroid medication, or if you're wanting further testing done, you'll benefit from doing some research ahead of the day and taking it along with you to back up your requests.

You'll find studies and evidence regarding the importance of full thyroid panel testing and the effectiveness of other medications for example, all over the internet but also on websites and in books such as this one (look at the back of this book). You can print them out, make notes on them, highlight important parts and take them along with you so you're prepared to fight your corner if needed.

## Body Language and Presentation

Keep in mind how your body language can help or hinder how assertive you are at your appointment. Breathe calmly and try not to get angry or frustrated. Remain mature and open for discussion and the doctor is more likely to take you and your concerns seriously. Talk directly at them, looking them in the eye if you can, ensuring that your confidence in being your own healthcare advocate is demonstrated.

## Consider Unexpected Outcomes

No one likes to think that after so much preparation and anxiety, a medical appointment might not go to plan. Take it from someone who had done months of research and calmly asked for a full thyroid panel to be tested and to try a different thyroid medication, and got shot down very patronisingly by a doctor who was not at all happy with my questions. I left that appointment upset and refused to see that particular GP at my surgery again. I somehow hadn't considered that they would refuse my suggestions and so I was totally unprepared and shocked.

Prepare yourself for various outcomes and how you would react so as not to be caught off guard, and remain realistic. Many doctors, especially in mainstream medicine, apply a 'one size fits all' approach to treating thyroid patients and refuse to acknowledge that so many of us are still unwell on standard medication therapy.

Underscoring all of this, please do remember that if you don't get on with a particular doctor or medical professional, or aren't happy with the treatment you receive, that you're entitled to find a new one. After all, no one knows your body as well as you do. Types of different medical professionals often seen by thyroid patients can be found in Chapter 7.

## Chapter Recap:

- It's normal to feel nervous about upcoming appointments, especially when you anticipate a doctor not listening to your concerns.
- It's a good idea to plan for appointments and go in prepared.
- Appointments may not always go to plan but don't lose hope.

# Chapter 9: How Work Can Be Affected with Thyroid Disease

*"My skills include reading a whole email without absorbing a single word." - Rachel Hill, The Invisible Hypothyroidism*

The effect that hypothyroidism can have on personal lives, social lives, work lives and more can be devastating. Whilst for some thyroid patients, they can go about living an almost normal life, such as that of their peers, for many others, their life is altered in huge ways.

As well as finding it harder to keep up with friends and family, and remain a social butterfly, house work, life admin and remaining in work can be very challenging.

I was diagnosed with autoimmune hypothyroidism at twenty-one years old and the workplace I was in at the time was luckily very supportive. Though I appreciate that this isn't the same for everyone.

My line manager and work colleagues witnessed me going through quite a tough time with testing, increasing symptoms and countless doctor's appointments, until the eventual diagnosis. By this time, I had been at that particular place of work for two years, originally starting as a healthy, bright eyed and bushy tailed apprentice.

They'd seen my decline and how I struggled to keep up with work like I used to; mentally *and* physically. For me, it presented in my reduced ability to make it into the office every day, with most weeks consisting of at least one missed day of work. At one point, I was practically bed-bound due to my poor physical health and felt lucky to have the bathroom just a few feet away from my bedroom, as that's all I needed all day whilst lying in bed feeling like a failure, with my flu-type symptoms and indescribable fatigue weighing my body down.

Other days, it was my mental health - anxiety and depression - also caused by my inadequately treated thyroid condition, that were the main reason I missed work. A sudden rush of panic as if something awful was going to happen but not being able to pinpoint *what* exactly, wasn't a rare occurrence. Panic attacks through the night. Night terrors. Not being able to stop crying whilst trying to get ready for work. I was a mental and emotional mess. My life was falling apart and so was I.

I was trying to deal with this the best I could behind closed doors as I felt too embarrassed to tell any friends or family about it, but it started spilling out into every corner of my life and I couldn't contain the effects of hypothyroidism on my life any longer. I was a wreck and a shell of my former self, and at only twenty-one years old, I thought '*this isn't normal*'.

I'm lucky that people in my workplace were so understanding at the time I really struggled to remain in work. Whenever I needed a day or two off, they just said *OK*. I wasn't made to feel like a bad person or employee, or judged for it. Colleagues would call or text me to check I was OK, and even the director of our area called me to give me some words of support and comfort. They let me know that they were there for me if I needed them, and my job was there for the days I could make it in. They pulled together and covered my work where they could, and on the days when I did come in, no big deal was made, which reduced anxiety over feeling embarrassed. Every few weeks, my manager would take me aside to talk about how I'd been doing, which reassured me that they cared. It was perfect, really. I couldn't have asked for anything more from them.

But I am well aware this isn't always the case for everyone. As knowledge about hypothyroidism among the general public is so poor anyway, workplaces often aren't aware of how much thyroid disease can cripple people. Doctors refusing to listen about how our inadequately treated hypothyroidism is affecting us and our work lives, are also causing a lot of harm, since this reiterates what our work colleagues and bosses may already think.

On a day when I did make it into work, it didn't exactly feel great, either. It didn't feel like a victory. It still felt like a loss. This is what a typical day was like for me:

*I go to bed at 8pm because I'm so unbelievably tired. I sleep pretty much straight through the night, maybe waking briefly during the night, but nothing to hugely disturb the amount of sleep I get, before my alarm goes off at 7am for work. That's 11 hours sleep. Yet I feel **more** tired than when I went to bed the night before. How is that possible?*

*I drag myself out of bed, force myself to have a shower, get dressed and make my way downstairs. All of this is hard because it's like I'm moving a dead weight. Putting on my trousers left me breathless and getting in the shower almost made me collapse. I'm also a bit dizzy, light headed and weak whilst doing these things, but I managed them, just.*

*As I make my way out the house, my legs are trying their best effort to stop me. Walking to work is draining every ounce of energy I do happen to have left after that shambles of a night's sleep. I feel sick, my heart is pounding and I'm having hot flushes. I'm scared I'm going to pass out but I keep going.*

*I get to work, and even though I have a sedentary office job, it's going to be a long day. The room feels freezing, even though everyone in the office doesn't feel the same. When someone opens a window or puts on a fan, my bones ache even more and it makes all my symptoms ten times worse. I struggle to get out of my chair and walk to the toilet. I struggle to get myself a drink or some food, if I even have the appetite for it. I struggle to type on my computer because my fingers individually hurt and my hands are weak.*

*When the phone rings, my heart stops with the shock of a loud noise. My reflexes are poor, and my arms are absolutely aching, with this heaviness that's like having weights tied to them, but I manage to answer the phone. I forget for a second what I'm supposed to say, then muster up a "Hello, Rachel speaking. How can I help you?" It comes out quiet and croaky. I feel drained already and it's only 9am. I'm exhausted in every inch of my body. My fingers are heavy and stiff.*

*For the rest of the day, it's a struggle to get anything done. I can't think straight, and even the simplest of tasks take 100 times more energy than if I weren't so fatigued. I answer the phone again later and forget completely what I'm supposed to say. I type an email and completely forget halfway through what I was going to type. Someone asked me if I wanted a cup of tea, and I can't compute what they've asked me. I have this mental block.*

*Mid-afternoon, I get a sudden slump where I feel even worse. My eyes are now heavier than ever, my blood pressure speeds up and things like back ache and headaches set in. They'll stay with me all day now.*

*After what feels like a twenty-hour day, I make my way home, barely even standing anymore. My body is punishing me without any reason. Yesterday was a normal day. I didn't overexert myself and I haven't done anything to deserve this struggle today.*

*I get through the front door and collapse on the sofa, just a few feet away from the door. I sleep for a couple hours, before waking up and seeing it's about 8pm, so I make my way to bed, and sleep for another 10-11 hours, maybe even more. If I'm lucky, I might manage to get some food and a drink. The fatigue can often make me feel sick, though.*

*I might sleep through the night, or tonight, despite feeling like I've ran a marathon, I toss and turn and can't get to sleep, knowing how awful I'm going to feel the next morning. I'm in despair and can't bare the next day.*

*My alarm goes off at 7am for work. I get up feeling more tired than when I went to bed the night before.*

*The same day unfolds.*

\* \* \*

Being suicidally depressed at the time added another layer to my struggle at work too. I had zero motivation, barely cared about keeping my job and couldn't concentrate on anything. All I could think about was how much physical and mental pain I was in, how drained I was all the time, how totally fed up I was, and basically, how I wanted it all to end.

How awful is it that even one person has to unnecessarily experience that?

I say *unnecessarily* as I'm sure you're aware by now, that we can indeed feel better and make a recovery back to a good quality of life. But for many, they still struggle with work and maintaining a good work life balance.

But please know that you are not alone. You're not lazy. You're not imagining it. But you *are* entitled to help and support.

## Maintaining Employment With Hypothyroidism

Whether you disclose your health conditions, mental and/or physical, to your employer is up to you. I personally find it much easier, when starting any new job, to disclose quite early on (though only once I've started a new job) that I live with X, Y and Z, and this is how they can affect me. Often, the perfect example will present itself for this, such as a doctor's appointment during work hours, opening the conversation between me and my employer.

I like to make my line manager and work colleagues aware of any extra support I may require, doctor's appointments or other health-related appointments which may pop up during work hours and generally just maintain open lines of communication. It makes it much easier to call in and tell my boss that I'm having a flare up day, if he already knows what a flare up consists of, because it causes me less anxiety and gives him a rough idea of when I'll be back at work.

For some of you, it may help to consider your role and if it's really suitable given your health situation. For example, are the hours ideal? I found that shift work never sat well with me, when my body runs so much better on routine.

I've come to recognise that my perfect number of working hours match a part time role. It wasn't an easy decision to come down from full time working to part time, but I did it gradually, until I reached the point that I saw a good balance.

This change in hours allowed me to have a much better work life balance as I was no longer spending all my time at home sleeping until I went back to work the next morning. I suddenly had time for myself, hobbies and socialising again. The balance was coming back.

Flexible working is also worth considering, so whether your employer is happy for you to move your working hours around to compensate for doctor's appointments or blood tests, or if they'll just let you have the hour or so out the office out of kindness, it can make your life a lot easier to have these agreements in place, so you're both aware of what works best for both your health and the business.

Working from home jobs are something that I've also considered in the past, as I've been in offices that are too cold, draughty and noisy, which, when having thyroid and adrenal dysfunction, were really hard to work in as I couldn't concentrate and perform at my optimal best.

Remote working can be great if you have mobility concerns with your hypothyroidism or your condition is just better managed in a familiar environment.

You should also consider the type of work you do, keeping in mind what you enjoy doing and find fulfilling. I've done some manual and hands-on work in the past, such as working as a care assistant in an elderly care home, as well as office work and I much prefer the latter. Wasting energy by being on my feet all day, not getting regular breaks and having the responsibility of caring for so many adults wasn't a great fit for my health. It was a lot of unneeded stress!

I tend to be most happy in an office environment that is a little calmer, has good routine and has more opportunities for me to take regular breaks to prevent becoming fatigued or more ill. I know many people who are guilty of not using their holiday allowance, either. Holiday days can not only be used for vacations, but for catching up with friends and family, day trips, duvet days or getting some personal tasks done at home. Utilise your holiday days.

You also need to be able to switch off from work, guarding plenty of time for yourself in the evenings and weekends (or whenever your non-work days are) for unwinding and enjoying your personal time.

When you can't switch off from work after leaving the office, this is a big warning sign that it's threatening to harm your health. Not switching off is a threat to your sleep quality and adrenal health, which, when consistent over a prolonged period of time, is a recipe for disaster when it comes to managing your thyroid condition. Avoid taking work home with you, checking emails outside of work hours and instead set *firm* boundaries.

Working can be more difficult for those with hypothyroidism and there's no shame in adjusting your work situation so that it allows you a better quality of life.

Having a good work-life balance is defined as feeling as if you have enough time and energy to devote to both your work and your personal activities separately. Not having this balance right can lead to feeling stressed, overworked and struggling physically as a result.

Juggling your hypothyroidism alongside working can feel difficult, especially if you have less energy levels than most people, doctors appointments to attend and need more time to recuperate outside of work, but considering the tips in this chapter can help to strike that balance.

## Speaking to Colleagues and Work Management

If you're feeling ready to talk to your workplace more about your condition, you could also arrange a fundraising activity at work to raise money for a thyroid charity, like a bake sale for example, and put up posters. People will ask what hypothyroidism is and that's your chance to raise awareness of it as a condition, but also how it affects you personally. Build good knowledge of this condition, so that people are more understanding and supportive. After all, we tend to spend so much of our time at work, the people we work with should know what we go through so they can best support us.

## Optimising Your Work Area

Some things that I have done in the past to make my workplace/area more hypothyroid appropriate include:

- Keeping a hot water bottle in my desk drawer - perfect for warming me up when feeling cold increases my brain fog and affects my ability to work as effectively.

- Keeping a blanket under my desk - for the same reason as above. Some colleagues have looked at me a bit strange in the past, but I really don't care if it helps me feel more comfortable!

- Taking my own stash of tea in - I've kept my own caffeine free, herbal and fruit teas in my desk at work before, as everyone else mostly drinks regular tea and coffee, and I avoid caffeine as it worsens adrenal fatigue and increases the chance of migraines.

- Having a water bottle on my desk - Keeping a water bottle on my desk reminds me to keep sipping water all day and stay hydrated which is so so important for a lot of reasons. I make sure to fill it up when I first arrive at work and then refill at lunch. I know I'm getting my goal amount of water before I've even headed home for dinner, then!

- Snacks - I love snacks. I often joke that they're the best meal of the day, so I try to keep some protein rich snacks in my desk at work for when I feel a wobbly blood sugar moment or pangs of hunger coming on. It's important to eat regularly.

**Important bits:**

If you feel discriminated at work, based on your health condition/s, you have a right to complain.

In the UK, if you think you've been unfairly discriminated against you should try to raise it with the person, your line manager, or even talk to Acas or Citizens Advice, or a trade union representative, if things cannot be sorted out informally. You might be able to take a claim to an employment tribunal for discrimination. Check if you can get legal aid to help with your legal costs if you think you've been discriminated against. Employers must follow the law on preventing discrimination at work.

If you're in another country, you can find information on discrimination at work online, but sadly I can't cover all countries in this little book! Just know that it isn't OK for you to be treated unfairly and you *do* have rights.

## Financial Support

Some of us with hypothyroidism can be so ill that we simply cannot work. I've been on that side of things and can't believe the ignorance when I hear other people insist that "hypothyroidism isn't a disability". Thyroid conditions, just like all other health conditions, can affect people on a scale. Whereas some may be able to work, others really do struggle. If you feel as if you need to claim financial support in the form of benefits for example, that is a completely personal decision.

Depending on the severity of your condition, such as how limiting your case of hypothyroidism is to your day to life, as well as if you have any other physical or mental health conditions or disabilities, then you *may* be entitled to financial support. If this applies to you, then get in contact with your local authority, have an honest and realistic conversation with your doctor and find out if you can receive any financial support. It may be that you require financial support whilst getting your thyroid health back on track and before you're able to slowly reintroduce work.

## Chapter Recap:

- Some people with thyroid conditions find that maintaining in employment can be difficult.

- Consider how suitable your line of work is and whether it is helping or hindering your recovery back to good health.

- Try to keep a good line of communication open.

- Consider ways of optimising your work environment and creating a good work-life balance.

- Do not feel ashamed if you struggle to work due to the effects of thyroid disease. Everyone is individual.

# Chapter 10: Grieving For Who You Were Before Hypothyroidism

*"You're going to be happy," said life. "But first, let me make you strong." - Unknown*

When you go through the diagnosis of a chronic illness, it's not uncommon to grieve. To grieve for the person you once were and the life you once had. I don't think it's unreasonable to say that most people who go from being a relatively healthy person to suddenly having a lifelong health condition, grieve. For some, they grieve for months, years or the rest of their lives, wondering what life they could have had, had they not gotten sick.

Before age twenty, which is when hypothyroidism symptoms really started to interfere with my life and become a big problem, I was an incredibly busy, active and driven person. I had completed 5k's, had a constantly full diary of social activities and events and prided myself on a spotless home. I was always on the go and people asked me how I did it. Looking back, I think *How on Earth did I do it realising now how unwell I was?!*

I would walk two miles to work and two miles back every day, before tidying the house and starting dinner. After dinner, I'd go to my dance class, go for a run or catch up on orders and product making for our small handmade jewellery business, which was run entirely in the evenings. I was ridiculously busy and able to maintain a full-time job, our own small business, the perfectly clean home, regular exercise sessions and a busy social life. I felt happy and fulfilled. I was a regular twenty-year-old loving life and embracing everything I could do. Before I got sick, I never felt tired and I bounced out of bed in the morning. I was the friend who organised everything and enjoyed doing so. I was a morning person. I was on top of everything.

My future looked bright as I imagined buying a house with my long-term partner one day and starting a family, and I was at the beginning of my career in event management. I imagined being a high-flying mum who did well in her career but was also hands-on with her children and was great at keeping an organised home; dinner on the table at five and having them washed and in bed, before putting my feet up for the evening. You know, the sort of thing you see in movies. I imagined a busy, organised life and loved the idea of it. I imagined that I would feel satisfied and had accomplished a lot, being good at what I did and as efficient as I was pre-illness.

But then, aged twenty, I started experiencing worsening symptoms; random leg cramps and spasms, migraines and a constant feeling of never waking up feeling refreshed, even after a lot of sleep. Eventually diagnosed with hypothyroidism and Hashimoto's, whilst I finally had an answer for how unwell I felt, my life was also about to change drastically.

I soon realised that I could no longer be the friend who made all the effort maintaining relationships and bearing all the responsibility for meetups and events. It wore me down and I didn't have the energy anymore. This was a blessing in disguise to realise that others needed to take on some responsibility for this part of our social lives, though.

It also dawned on me that I may struggle to conceive and carry children to full-term one day due to hypothyroidism, and that I would need a lot of extra help in raising a family, due to my newly diagnosed chronic illnesses affecting energy levels and more. I wouldn't be as efficient a parent as I once assumed. Caring for someone else suddenly seemed really scary when I was now needing a lot of help myself. Some days my partner was having to aid me up the stairs, in the shower, when getting dressed and more. The thought of being like this but also pregnant or a mother seemed impossible. My dreams were shattered.

I also had to accept that I couldn't be as active as I once was, until my health steadily improved again. Walking ten miles a week, playing badminton, running and dance lessons every Monday, were just not doable anymore. Not with my health like this. I needed to slow down.

I had to accept that my house wasn't always going to be as clean and tidy as it used to be because I had to learn to prioritise my energy and I quite frankly didn't have the energy anymore to spend time everyday cleaning like I used to. But again, this was a blessing in disguise because I soon learnt that a spotless home wasn't the most important thing.

I realised that my body wasn't as strong and capable as it once was and that some days I would be forgetful, achy and fatigued beyond words, also catching illnesses easier and taking longer to recover from them, compared to other people my age. I started missing a lot of time off work and I began living in a world of brain fog and low energy.

I had to learn to mourn the person I was before I developed hypothyroidism, as well as the life I assumed I would have. Everything was going to be different now. But how do you even begin to move on? Often, we have to get through the period of grieving, with all five stages: denial, anger, bargaining, depression and acceptance, before we're able to really start healing.

As I write this book, I have been diagnosed for almost three and a half years now, and yes, I've accepted how my life and even *I* have changed, with the adjustments and many ups and downs that living with hypothyroidism can bring, but I do sometimes get frustrated and miss who I once was and what I was able to do without much of a thought. Especially on bad health days. But you have to move on past those thoughts or you end up torturing yourself with pointless 'what ifs'.

Ninety-nine percent of my days now aren't ruled by my thyroid condition anymore, but I'm still going to have flare ups every now and again. That's just realistic.

Whilst it's true that you can indeed live a full life with hypothyroidism (and I hope my book has taught you this), it doesn't tend to come without learning to adapt and adjust to now having a chronic illness. Whether that involves learning how to manage your energy levels because they're no longer limitless, making dietary changes, implementing a better sleeping schedule or one of the many other interventions I've mentioned in this book, they demonstrate that you need to make adaptations and adjustments to help you live that full life. They demonstrate that you have to welcome in this new way of living and let go of what you used to have. Basically, *grieve*.

I initially missed being able to work-out a few times a week, building muscle and tone, the buzz it gave me when I surpassed a personal best, the adrenaline rush and how invigorating it felt to run and do as much physical activity as I used to. However, I realised and accepted that my body didn't like this form of exercise post-thyroid issue, and so have supplemented it for others that help instead of *hindering* my health. These days, I do three dance classes a week and walk for around an hour every day. Running may be a thing of the past but by making this adjustment, my health has been able to recover. And I love that I've found a new (and more enjoyable) fitness regimen.

I sometimes miss just being able to do what I like without running out of energy, as I never had to plan my energy usage like I sometimes do now. However, what I do not miss is blaming myself for failing to have the energy to complete my work out, as my hypothyroidism was developing and I wasn't yet diagnosed. I do not miss beating myself up and telling myself I was lazy. I do not miss forcing my body to try and keep up with the exercise routine despite feeling so unwell.

I have learnt to appreciate the small things; sure, I'm still a bit of a neat freak, but I'm able to leave a pot to be washed tomorrow and the laundry can be ironed another day, instead of freaking out over it and always being on the move, cleaning and tidying. With my 'new life' of having hypothyroidism, I am encouraged to prioritise rest more, which gives me more time to enjoy self-care, relaxing and winding down, and even having a cuddle with my husband in front of the TV.

Having a thyroid condition has been a blessing in disguise really because it has encouraged me to put a lot of things into perspective and realise what is and isn't important. When life moves as fast as it does in this day and age, it's easy to try and keep up with everyone else but the truth is, you have to go at your own pace otherwise you'll never heal.

My life is different and always will be since being diagnosed with thyroid disease, but I have embraced this now and instead of thinking about what it has stolen from me, I think about what it has taught me, and how much of a better person I am because of it. It has shaped who I am today. I have grieved for the person I once was and the life I once had, but I have accepted that my life was never destined to be the way I imagined before, and now, I have to strive to do the best with what I've got.

Hypothyroidism and Hashimoto's do not have to feel like a death sentence. You *can* still live a good quality, full life with hypothyroidism but to get there, accepting your new life and all the adjustments is crucial in you moving forward. Learning to accept your new life and the way everything has changed is *liberating*. Sure, you'll need to adjust, adapt and learn how to do some things again, but you'll figure it all out.

Even though my quality of life is really good these days, my life still looks very different to how it did before I got sick. I followed all the information I've presented to you in this book and then made some extra adjustments based on my own individual requirements and now, I can say that I enjoy life again and my thyroid condition doesn't rule it. Instead, I manage my thyroid condition. And by doing that I've taken back my life and learnt to let go of what it was pre-hypothyroidism.

Trying to look at having hypothyroidism in a more positive light can be difficult, but it has helped me to get through the grieving stage and accept my new life with the condition.

For example, it has taught me to be a stronger person. As soon as I had the symptoms of hypothyroidism, I researched about it and soon learnt that I had to accept I was in this for the long-run and so I was going to have to give it my best shot. When I felt at my absolute worst, on

Levothyroxine, I had a few months of despair, of not being able to accept that I would feel this way forever, and then something clicked. I realised I didn't have to. I became strong in my ability to push for answers and keep on going, because the alternative, to live a rubbish quality of life, just wasn't an option.

It has also taught me to look after myself better and be an active participant in my own healthcare. I already exercised a lot and ate a healthy diet, but I learnt that I could do too much and actually cause more harm than good. I was expecting a lot from my body and needed to slow down and listen to it. Through being an active participant in my own healthcare and embracing being my own thyroid advocate, I started to take my health back in to my own hands, changing thyroid medication, exploring other problems and arranging further testing. I taught myself how to interpret my test results and what I should be aiming for. I grew in confidence and independence. I realised that the thyroid patients who get better are often the ones who pay attention to their own treatment; not leave it all up to a doctor.

Hypothyroidism has also taught me that sometimes I need to ask for help and that's OK too. I don't have to do it all on my own. I used to have very high expectations, unrealistic expectations, for myself, that I would never drift from. I expected a lot from myself and was a perfectionist in every way possible. Now, I understand that it's OK to not get every task done each day, because I am only human. I'm human with a health condition that can get in the way at times. I now know when to ask for help and get other people to pull their weight, too. I've learnt how to strike a balance in life.

My health conditions taught me that we can empower ourselves with books, resources and other thyroid patients' experiences, in order to gain invaluable knowledge. From this, I am more knowledgeable, not just about thyroid and endocrine problems, but also about doctors, the healthcare system, and reading lab work in general. I've become more mature and wiser.

Hypothyroidism has developed my knowledge and through that I have learnt things I never knew I could. Who knew the girl that struggled to stay awake in science classes at school would go on to know so much about thyroid health?

It has also taught me that connecting with other thyroid patients can be invaluable to our own recovery. I have met many new people and made a lot of friends through having hypothyroidism. How crazy is that?! Some people already in my life had hypothyroidism too, but I didn't even know until I shared my diagnosis with them. Other friends, I have made through my online support group, or through other social media platforms I have used. Fellow thyroid patients are often the only people who truly understand my experiences and struggles. As a community, we help each other.

Through all the devastation that hypothyroidism can cause, I like to remember the positive things it has done for me. I do wonder what my life would have been like had I never developed it, or perhaps if I had developed it later on in life (as twenty is considered to be quite young to develop a thyroid condition), but I don't think I would be as good a version of myself I am today, if I hadn't. I am stronger, wiser and more compassionate.

Perhaps keeping a note of any positive changes you feel going through this experience, once you start recovering your health, would help you to accept your new life with hypothyroidism, as it did mine. You may be surprised.

## Chapter Recap:

- Many of us feel a sense of grief after being diagnosed with a health condition such as a thyroid condition.
- Your life may change but it's not necessarily always for the worse.
- Looking for the positive changes (however hard this can seem) is helpful.

# Chapter 11: Dear Friends and Family

*"If you love someone, let them nap." - Rachel Hill, The*
*Invisible Hypothyroidism*

Those of us with hypothyroidism may want to share the next chapter with loved ones.

Friends and family of a thyroid patient, your role in the care and management of their chronic health condition is pivotal. Your support, acknowledgement and understanding of all that they go through and how they make their journey back to good health is crucial in their recovery. This chapter is specifically for you.

One of my most popular ever articles has been the open letter I wrote to those who know someone with hypothyroidism. Shared and read thousands of times already and also republished across other websites, I couldn't *not* include it in my book.

This open letter was written with the aim of giving those around us a better understanding of what it is we go through and how they can help us, when living with hypothyroidism. I promise it's worth the read and your friend or family member with the condition will be more grateful than you'll ever imagine.

## An Open Letter to Those Who Know Someone with Hypothyroidism

Hello friend, family member, work colleague or doctor of someone who lives with an underactive thyroid or hypothyroidism.

You know someone very strong, battling an often-difficult disease.

If you're not a medical professional, you're probably wondering what exactly an underactive thyroid or hypothyroidism is, or how it affects someone who lives with it, so I'll do my best to explain it as simply as possible.

You've likely already heard some things about it, for example that it is an excuse people use for being overweight. But this is far from what it really does to someone. In reality, hypothyroidism does so much more to its host. It hurts when we see people use the term "thyroid problem" as code to describe someone who is overweight. It also belittles the condition. It's so much worse than just weight gain, although this is still a legitimate symptom.

The thyroid gland is located in the neck and its hormones are required for every cell and function of the body. An underactive thyroid means just that; it's under active. It's slow and sluggish and not performing properly, meaning a slow metabolism that causes weight gain and very little energy, as well as lots of other symptoms. The same goes for those who are hypothyroid through having no thyroid gland at all.

For the thyroid gland to function properly, we need the right amount of thyroid hormones in our bodies. If we don't have these, it affects our energy levels and lots of other things, especially things you probably don't even think about. For example, sleep cycles, body temperature, alertness, thinking clearly, appetite and fertility, to name just a few.

Hypothyroidism is most commonly caused by an autoimmune disease, such as Hashimoto's Thyroiditis or Graves' Disease. Sometimes it is caused by having treatment for hyperthyroidism (an overactive thyroid) or having had treatment for thyroid cancer. The treatment often used for these, radioactive iodine treatment or a thyroidectomy, can result in the patient becoming hypothyroid. So, any of these could have caused the person you know to have the condition.

You may even know another person with hypothyroidism, who takes medication for it and is seemingly OK, but this isn't the same for all thyroid patients. Actually, a lot of thyroid patients find it's not easily treated and controlled. The other person you know may not have told you the full extent of how it affects them, either.

Hypothyroidism can cause mental health conditions like depression and anxiety, as well as physical symptoms like loss of hair, brain fog, aches and pains throughout the body, constipation, an increase or decrease in blood pressure and even scary heart palpitations and loss of appetite, to name just a few.

You can imagine that a lack of sleep, or needing to sleep lots but actually not feeling any better when we do, may make the simplest of everyday tasks difficult or impossible for a thyroid patient.

The best way I can describe hypothyroidism symptoms is by comparing it to the flu. The fatigue and aches are very similar. You know how frustrated, fed-up and useless you feel when you're ill and have things to do? That's how it can be to have hypothyroidism. Except we have no choice but to work, run a family, house, maintain a social life (or at least try to) and try to maintain a positive attitude towards life.

Combine it with all of these symptoms here:

- Constipation
- Depression
- Slow movements, speech and thoughts
- Itchy and/or sore scalp
- Muscle cramps
- Dry and tight feeling skin
- Brittle hair and nails

- Pain, numbness and a tingling sensation
- Irregular periods or heavy periods
- Brain fog/confusion/memory problems
- Migraines
- Hoarse voice
- A puffy-looking face
- Thinned or partly missing eyebrows
- Poor stamina
- Long recovery period after any activity
- Arms feeling like dead weights after activity
- Inability to exercise, or withstand certain exercises
- Tendency to be overly emotional
- Inability to tolerate cold – cold hands and feet
- Poor circulation
- High or rising cholesterol
- Acid reflux
- Swollen legs that impede walking
- Difficulty standing on feet
- Joint stiffness and pain
- Fertility issues

and you get the picture of what it's like.

So, you can imagine that sometimes, thyroid patients living with these have to cancel plans last minute, through no fault of their own. When they have plans to do something, they tend to look forward to it, as it can take their mind off their health condition or make them feel like they're taking back some control. So, if they then have to cancel on you due to hypothyroid symptoms and struggles, you can imagine how devastated they likely feel. The next time you think they might be making up excuses, being lazy or being a cop-out, please realise that when this is their life, they have no real control and they are not to blame.

**We didn't *choose* to have thyroid disease.**

Thyroid patients are often not easily understood by those around them. We're made to feel like this condition isn't a big thing to live with as it is often not taken seriously. Most people think it's an easily treated condition, when in reality, it is none of those things for many patients. We're not hypochondriacs, it really does cause lots of symptoms.

Yes, for some thyroid patients they do OK on standard thyroid medication but for many, they still struggle.

Even some of our friends, family and work colleagues (this could be you) overlook how serious it is, and how detrimental it can be to our lives. Even some doctors look at it like this. Not all, but a lot. A lot more than we should have to experience when fighting to regain some quality of life.

Many patients struggle to actually get diagnosed for years, with doctors brushing it off as depression, chronic fatigue syndrome or fibromyalgia, among other things. Doctors regularly misdiagnose hypothyroidism. Even when we are diagnosed and started on medication, we often find it takes some time to feel better, or that doctors will not consider another type of medication if the first one they try doesn't work for us. A lot of us even have to turn to going private for our healthcare or sourcing the medication ourselves. So, don't assume that your friend, family member or work colleague is 'OK now they've got medication for it'. Instead, please ask us.

Can you imagine how lonely we feel sometimes? Alone in our struggles and feeling like no one understands?

What we would like from you is to be the person who understands what we're going through, and that even though it's not a well-recognised disease, it is a real, difficult, life-changing condition. It often destroys, changes and alters lives forever.

The best thing you can do is to be there for your friend, family member or work colleague who has this disease; all we need you to do is listen, and learn about the struggles and challenges we face. We don't expect you to know everything, but to be understanding and sympathetic when we are struggling. You could help the thyroid patient in your life do as much as possible to improve their health, be it encourage them to seek out a doctor who will listen, or do research with them to learn more about how they can help themselves feel better.

When they read a new book, read it with them. Thyroid brain fog can make us forget a lot of what we read! Encourage them to pick up new thyroid books. Be the person who helps them to find time for rest, self-care and time to enjoy what they love doing most. It might be helpful for you to read about other patients' experiences, too. Ask us if we need help with anything and ask us how we've been feeling. It's good to know someone cares.

If you live with a thyroid patient, don't expect too much from them in daily life. I'm not saying that all thyroid patients are incapable of doing anything, far from it actually, but rather that you shouldn't expect them to do as much as they used to. Instead, let them rediscover their limits and stamina.

You may have to take up more of the housework and take initiative on things that they used to be in charge of in order to help. Tell them when they've done enough for the day and encourage them to rest. Bring them drinks, run them a bath, or simply ask if they need help getting up the stairs or putting their shoes on. Go with them to doctor appointments and help them get the right treatment for them. Encourage them to find online support groups and networks to meet others also living with the disease. Often, experience and advice can be shared among patients, which is invaluable to helping make the condition that little bit easier to live with.

Something as simple as reading this letter, means the world to us. It means a lot that you want to understand our situation and help us, or at least be someone we can talk and rant to, and rely on to listen to us when we're having a hard day.

\* \* \*

## The Spoon Theory: Understanding How Your Loved One's Energy Levels Work

Something else that can be really useful to know about as someone who has a friend or family member with hypothyroidism, is understanding and applying the spoon theory.

My husband describes the moment that I shared this simple analogy with him, as a light bulb switching on. He could understand more easily how my energy levels and depletions work and that really helped him to help me, the thyroid patient.

### So, what is the spoon theory?

The spoon theory is a metaphor those with a disability, chronic illness and/or autoimmune disease, for example, use to explain the reduced amount of energy available for activities of daily living and tasks. And a 'spoonie', is someone with a chronic illness, who needs to watch their 'spoons'.

### Let me explain what the spoon theory is.

The idea of the spoon theory, by Christine Miserandino, explains how those living with disability or chronic illness have a limited amount of energy.

The idea is that many people with a disability or chronic illness must carefully plan their daily activities to use their energy wisely, while most people with better health or who do not have a disability, do not need to worry about running out of energy.

'Spoons' are a unit of measurement used to track how much energy a person has throughout the day. Imagine you start the day with a certain number of 'spoons'. You need to get through the day without using them all too early on.

Each activity requires a certain number of spoons (such as having a shower, walking to work, making dinner), and spoons will only be replaced as the person rests. If you run out of spoons (energy), you have no choice but to rest until your spoons are replenished.

For example, you could start each day with ten spoons and tasks just as showering or bathing require two spoons, and walking for half an hour requires six. Those of us with limited energy reserves have to work out what activities we can afford to do each day, so as not to run out of spoons (energy) and be left exhausted.

You can also end up going in to the next day's allocation of spoons by overexerting yourself, and then take longer to replenish them (your energy levels).

As other people without a disability or chronic illness do not feel the impact of spending spoons for mundane tasks such as bathing and getting dressed, they may not realise the amount of energy used by those who *do* need to plan their energy usage just to get through the day. They do not tend to have a limited amount of energy, as most daily tasks could never get close to exhausting them, unlike those with hypothyroidism for example.

Even those who have their hypothyroidism well managed tend to be more at risk of over exhausting and expecting too much of ourselves, compared to other people. Risking depleting our energy levels quickly.

As someone who knows a Spoonie, you should be aware of how they manage their energy levels and look for signs that they may be doing too much. Offering to help with certain tasks and saving us some spoons can mean we're actually able to do more *with you*.

My husband taking on more of the housework for example means I don't run out of energy as quickly as I used to, resulting in me napping a lot. Now I have more energy thanks to him helping me protect my spoons, which means I can spend more time with him doing the things we love.

## What Not to Say to Someone with Hypothyroidism

The below comments can cause people living with hypothyroidism to feel very alone, misunderstood, misjudged and avoid turning to people for help and support in the future, so they can be very detrimental.

This list hasn't been created to moan at you, the loved one, but to educate you so that you're able to help the thyroid patient in your life, as the support you can provide will aid their recovery a lot.

You may even be as shocked to hear these as we often are!

### 1. "You just need a good night's sleep."

Unfortunately, this just isn't how it works. Believe us, we've tried sleeping lots and we're not cured yet! And if you live with someone with hypothyroidism, you've probably noticed how much they sleep and how little difference it seems to make. In fact, we're so fatigued that we often sleep more than anyone else we know. It's frustrating!

Thyroid hormone directly controls and affects energy levels, which means that fatigue is one of the most commonly complained of symptoms with the condition. We are easily tired and often feel tired all the time, scarcely waking up feeling refreshed. The best way I can describe it is *every-second-I'm-consciously-having-to-keep-each-eyelid-open* tired. It's *I'm-scared-to-blink-or-I'll-fall-asleep* tired. It's exhaustion past the point of exhaustion.

## 2. "You've got medicine now, so you must be fine."

Not necessarily and this is a very big misconception. Unfortunately, it can take months or even years for people to get their thyroid medication right.

Since a lot of doctors aren't usually very helpful when it comes to trying different medication options to see what works for each patient, it can be a real upwards battle at times. Most tend to have a 'one medication works for all' approach which is very unhelpful. And even when we do get our thyroid medication right, we can also have other conditions that have developed because of the thyroid not being adequately treated for quite some time.

This includes vitamin deficiencies, adrenal problems, mental health conditions and digestive issues to name just a few. So, don't just assume we're OK once we're put on thyroid medication, as it's usually just the beginning! We're happy to talk to you about how we're doing and how our current medication is working.

## 3. "Be patient."

Being told to give the thyroid medication time to work can be frustrating. If we become a little impatient, frustrated or fed up, please bear with us. We've probably had a long battle with getting this diagnosis in the first place, so allow us to feel a little impatient. Don't you feel impatient waiting for the *us* you remember before hypothyroidism, to fully return?

### 4. "Just eat less and exercise more!"

As the metabolism is often slowed in hypothyroidism, we can have symptoms associated with a slow metabolism, such as cold intolerance, extreme tiredness and weight gain. We may gain weight and cannot control it. We also struggle to then lose it. Some even diet and force unhealthy exercise regimens and end up gaining more weight.

Only when our thyroid hormone levels are corrected, thus correcting our metabolic function, do we have a chance of losing excess weight and stop gaining it at all. Not to mention that most of us don't have the energy to move any more than we already do, due to the slow metabolism. Over exercising can also make you *more* hypothyroid.

### 5. "It's all in your head. You just need to let it go."

My own doctor told me this when I visited him time and time again complaining of my initial thyroid medication not helping at all. Needless to say, I haven't seen that doctor since, as I was so frustrated and I found one who does now listen and has got me on the medication I need to feel well.

### 6. "You're so hormonal!"

Please don't judge us because of our health condition. Please don't assume anything we say that you disagree with, is because our 'crazy thyroid hormones' make our moods and emotions go up and down.

We can be mad, annoyed or irritated for legitimate reasons. Maybe we're fed up with battling this health condition, but don't assume that it's just because of our thyroid hormones being off.

## 7. "You have this condition because of ___"

Insert 'not wearing a coat when you go out', 'your bad diet', 'not eating enough fruit and veg' etc. here. Sure, those things won't help your health, but hey, it doesn't cause thyroid problems either!

## 8. "The thyroid doesn't even do anything."

This not only belittles what we're going through, but it also makes you look very uninformed. Sure, I didn't even know where the thyroid gland was when I was first diagnosed! But don't assume it doesn't do anything. It actually does a lot of important stuff. The thyroid gland produces hormones needed for every process and every cell of the body, so when this goes wrong, a lot of other stuff does too!

## What is Helpful to Say to Someone with Hypothyroidism

These examples are instead much more helpful and will help to strengthen your mutual understanding of the condition and experience.

## 1. "How are you doing?"

This simple question shows you care about us and how we're doing, and that you understand we may have a bit of a battle with getting well again. It's nice to know that someone cares and we often like to talk about it with others so we don't feel alone. Let us get things off our chest too, it's very healthy and can help us to process the change in our lives.

## 2. "Can I do anything to help?"

Most commonly, you won't be able to do an awful lot, but we can benefit from you helping us with errands, housework or even an ear to listen. There's not a great deal our friends, family and work colleagues can do other than to be understanding of our condition and be open minded, but we'll rarely turn down the offer of a cup of tea and a chat.

Little things mean a lot to us when we're struggling. We're really grateful for those little things.

## 3. "What has worked for you?"

Treating and managing hypothyroidism is often not as simple as you'd think, so we tend to have to try quite a few medications, lifestyle adjustments and more until we find what works for us. This means lots of book reading, internet searching and maybe even numerous visits to different doctors and health practitioners. It can be stressful, upsetting and really testing at times, so we'd love to share with you what we've learnt and what we're going through. It's comforting to know you understand that it isn't a simple one-cure-fits-all disease.

## 4. "I respect your opinions/I support your choices."

Try not to dismiss us when we say that we know something isn't right, or that a particular treatment isn't working for us.

Respect us for doing our own research, and respect our opinions. Let us share our findings with you. Explore with us our ideas and acknowledge that we're entitled to our own thoughts, too. Support our choices to make changes to our health regimen if we feel it's the best thing for us. Really just try to understand and listen to us. This one is most important for partners of thyroid patients.

## 5. "You're looking well."

If we're looking better, brighter, happier, healthier, then let us know! It's reassuring to know that our hard work at getting ourselves better is paying off. We often lack motivation and many of us battle with mental health conditions that make it difficult to stay positive. Some praise every now and then and reminders that we're making progress can go a long way to give us the boost we need to carry on progressing in our journey to feeling better.

## 6. "How is the book you're reading?"

See us reading a thyroid book? A study or some research? Health magazine? A blog? Articles online maybe? Ask us what it's about, if it's any good and what we may have learnt from it. It's nice to see some interest from those around us and we'd like to share what we read with you too.

## 7. "You need to try another doctor."

If we're going back again and again to the same doctor and getting nowhere with feeling better, you may need to encourage us to seek out another. And another. And another. Until we find one who will listen to us and work *with* us. We can feel intimidated or worried to make the change, but it's important for our health that we do so. Again, your support is going to be key in us making progress with our health.

## 8. "Keep on going. You will feel well again."

When this condition and all its related problems get too much for us, we need to be reminded that we must keep on going. Often, facing the idea of spending the rest of our lives feeling so unbelievably ill, is enough to make someone very depressed and/or anxious. People with hypothyroidism can get better, and although it's not always easy, it is possible. It absolutely is. They just need gentle nudges and direction on where to go, at times. Help them to help themselves.

*  *  *

My other book builds on this chapter. *You, Me and Hypothyroidism: When Someone You Love Has Hypothyroidism* is for the friends, family and partners of those with hypothyroidism.

# Chapter 12: Dear Hypothyroid Patient

*"I know you're tired, but you have to keep on going."* - *Rachel Hill, The Invisible Hypothyroidism*

Dear hypothyroid patient,

Through having an underactive thyroid/hypothyroidism, you may feel lost, frustrated and lonely. At times, you may even feel fed up.

But you will also become stronger, more independent and protective of your health.

You don't need me to tell you that living with hypothyroidism and all its related conditions and issues isn't easy. The fatigue is overwhelming and the aches and pains are just awful. It's frustrating when your brain tells you to do something but your bodily physically *won't do it.*

Your mind may also start to fail you, brain fog making things harder to comprehend, and forgetfulness and confusion becoming parts of your everyday life. Feeling like you're failing your friends and family may be common and feeling as if you can't keep up with housework or your job can make you feel low. A failure. *An adult who can't adult.*

But you are not a failure, you are stronger than you give yourself credit for.

It takes someone strong to get up day after day, feeling like you have the flu, except it never gets better and never goes away. Getting out of bed is difficult enough, but running a family, having a job and generally trying to muddle on through life with such an often debilitating chronic health condition, is nigh on impossible. You're not a failure, you accomplish *so much* each and every day.

Our mental health often suffers too and let me tell you that it is *not* all in your head. Whether your doctor believes you or not. Depression and anxiety are common with hypothyroidism, yes, but not all of your symptoms can be pinned on these. That overwhelming fatigue, joint pain, muscle pain, headaches, acid reflux, brain fog, slowness, hoarse voice, weight gain, cold intolerance and so much more is valid. You are valid.

You will no doubt go through a tough diagnosis of hypothyroidism; it actually often takes ages for people to finally receive the diagnosis. And when you get it, you'll probably feel a sense of relief – a *reason* for feeling so rubbish. You're not a hypochondriac.

But if your symptoms don't go away as easily as the doctor's say they should, I promise you, you are not mad. You are not wrong to question the standard of care you are receiving and you should most definitely become your own thyroid advocate.

What I mean by that is taking back control of your own health, picking up books, digging for answers and fighting for better treatment. Stand up for yourself. You're entitled to a good standard of care. Ensure you are educated on your thyroid condition and know what you need to do to improve it, so you can gain a better quality of life. It's *so* important to take responsibility for your health. You need to embrace it.

What others without hypothyroidism (including doctors) often fail to realise, is that we put up with an *awful lot*. Along with the endless symptoms and related health conditions having hypothyroidism brings, we are often misrepresented, with a lot of the general public thinking that *'thyroid condition'* is just a term used when you need an excuse for being overweight. A lot of people don't even know where the thyroid gland is located in the body, let alone how debilitating it is and how much it can affect someone's life.

And so you shouldn't feel guilty for cancelling plans. You're not being unreliable – your body is. When you can't make it into work or all you've accomplished today is getting out of bed, you owe nobody an apology. You're entitled to feel the way you feel and you need to take care of yourself. When someone says that *'others have it worse'*, it can be detrimental in the way that that thyroid patient may no longer open up to someone when they need to, and why should they feel like what they're going through is any less relevant? We're all entitled to feel the way we feel. Don't compare your plight to others'.

You might feel alone sometimes and like no one else understands, which I get. When you're going through a vastly misunderstood, often not spoken about health condition that wreaks havoc on your body, mind and life, you can feel as if no one else 'gets it' or cares. Sat at home alone again, friends out having fun, you wonder what exactly the point in life is, these days. Thinking about how your life would have been, had you not developed a thyroid condition, you go through the five stages of grief: denial, anger, bargaining, depression and then, hopefully, acceptance. But this can take some time to reach.

For a while, you may be thinking *'why me? What did I do to deserve this?'*

You didn't do anything. You were simply unlucky. But you've got to move on from that.

Let me tell you, though, you are not alone in how you feel. You may feel lonely, but alone you are not. There is a whole community of thyroid patients out there with whom you can connect with. Whether you want to rant, confide in or ask for support, hypothyroid patients are among the most caring and supportive. *We understand.* We get you.

What I most importantly want to tell you, is that you can get better, though. You can. And you deserve to. Everyone deserves a good quality of life. Thyroid conditions often aren't easy to treat and manage, but with some research, digging, trial and error, you will find what medication works for you, any supplements, lifestyle changes and new approaches. But you've got to embrace being your own advocate, as I've already explained.

There will be better days, but you have to find the drive within you to get there. Never questioning your doctor or treatment and accepting that your quality of life and health is poor, will never reap results. I understand that motivation can be absent with hypothyroidism, I've been there, but hold on to the hope of being able to play physical games with your children again before collapsing on the sofa. Hold on to the hope of being able to *enjoy* your work, being an adult and everyday life. When things don't feel like a conscious effort anymore.

You have to keep on going, even when you don't think you can anymore. When tears are streaming down your face and you're sat in a deep dark hole you just can't see yourself ever climbing out of, you just have to keep on swimming. It's not going to be easy, but is it going to be worth it? Oh yes.

You're stronger than you believe. You're amazing.

You've got this and I *do* understand.

Rachel, The Invisible Hypothyroidism.

# Chapter 13: We're Cheering You On

*"Don't be ashamed of your story. It will inspire others."* - *Unknown*

Living with hypothyroidism and Hashimoto's is not always a straight journey. Once you get those symptoms, that diagnosis, the medication, your life changes forever and it can become a rollercoaster of ups and downs, highs and lows. Piecing back together the jigsaw puzzle of your thyroid health is hardly ever easy, but is it worth it? Oh yes.

I soon learnt what I hope you have also through reading my book; that you have to embrace becoming your own thyroid advocate and start educating yourself in order to move forward.

You will inevitably come up against bumps in the road, brick walls and tornados that really test your ability to keep on going, so what do you do? You climb over the bumps, smash through the walls and weather the tornados, because your story isn't going to end there.

You have to keep putting one foot in front of the other. Read books, studies, blogs, websites. Talk to other patients, medical practitioners and thyroid advocacies. Implement changes and take every trial and error with all you've got. Because you will reach that place of good health one day, you just have to keep on going.

## I Believe in You

In 2015, just after my diagnosis, autoimmune hypothyroidism plunged me into a deep, dark place called depression and I'm not ashamed to say that I was suicidal. Heck, of course I shouldn't feel ashamed. It's a reality that so many thyroid patients face, due to the inadequate thyroid treatment we so often receive. The doctors who left me there should be ashamed, if anyone, not me.

I was in physical and mental pain 24/7, I was beyond constantly fatigued and I had next to no quality of life. I couldn't bear the thought of living this way for the rest of my life and I felt my life had been unfairly ripped away from me. I was twenty-one and felt like a ninety-one-year-old, but every doctor told me I was 'fine' and that it was all in my head. I was made to feel crazy and made out to be a hypochondriac, which only made my mental health and physical health worse. At this time, I was of course inadequately treated for my hypothyroidism as Levothyroxine wasn't helping me and I hadn't realised there were many other pieces to this thyroid jigsaw puzzle yet.

It was difficult to find hope of a better quality of life when I was in this place, and so I would often have periods of doing OK and then periods of feeling really hopeless and fed up again. I tried, I really tried to have a 'positive mindset' but it didn't work. Not for longer than a couple of days anyway, because no matter how 'positively' I tried to think, I was always faced with the stark reality that I had a chronic illness for the rest of my life. It was difficult to get myself out of the hole of depression and I tried all sorts. But do you know what helped me on my way? Hope.

As soon as I discovered hope that I could get better, I started to see the light at the end of the tunnel again. Hope for me came in the form of books, online websites and blogs, podcasts and of course other thyroid patients' stories.

Hearing real people say that they got better and learnt to manage their hypothyroidism was more powerful than anything.

Of course, this didn't cure me of all my problems in a blink; it took a lot of tests, trying different medications, different types of doctors, supplements and persistence to make improvements in my mental and physical health. But these stories from others gave me hope in the darkest of times and I hope that my story in this book gives you a solid dose of hope too.

And so, when difficult seas come along to test my sailing ability again, as I've come to learn that living with my thyroid condition is an ongoing, always up and down affair, I remind myself that there are better days ahead, but for now, I just need to weather the storm. When I am in a flare up phase of my health conditions, I remind myself of the good health days and that I'll experience them once again.

And I wanted to share this with you because as you go out into the world and hopefully, after reading this book, begin your journey to good thyroid health with all the guidance and reassurance contained here within, I want you to be sure that you can keep on going when you hit the bumps and feel like you can't continue. Because you really can.

I'm living proof of someone who was once in an incredibly dark, hopeless place with this disease and if I can make it out, you certainly can too. Just remember that there's a whole thyroid community out there cheering you on.

## "Heard" a Poem by Rachel Hill, The Invisible Hypothyroidism

You wake up feeling more tired than when you went to bed
You have to cancel on your friends again and they say
you're a mess.
People at work have absolutely no clue
What it is exactly you're going through.

Waking up feeling like you have the worst kind of flu
But with poor mental health and weight gain added too.

Doctor after doctor tells you you're OK
But in your mind you know there's something else at play.

Your partner thinks you're lazy and dismisses your concerns
Family should understand but their lack of it burns.

You wonder 'Is this the new normal? How I'm going to
feel for the rest of my life?'
The thought of it kills the last of you inside.

'What happened to the person I once was?
The dreams I had, the plans I made
And a life not ruled by feeling lost?'

You feel alone, not listened to and batted down
But please know that there are others like you around.

We're also feeling just the way you do
And just how you need our support
We could do with yours too.

Together we can battle to win back our lives
Our health and our dreams
Let's take the dive.

We can empower each other to owe it to who we once were
So unite and scream out *"We deserve to be heard!"*

# Tests You May Need and Where To Order Them

*"If you want better, you need to make the changes."* – Rachel Hill, *The Invisible Hypothyroidism*

As a thyroid patient, the below blood tests are recommended to get the full picture of what's going on with your health. If you still have symptoms, despite being on thyroid medication, you can explore these. If you feel in good health, it is a good idea to monitor these regularly.

You may have to repeatedly ask your doctor or try a few different types of medical professionals (see Chapter 7) before you find one who will check all of them. Alternatively, many thyroid patients are ordering their own tests online which could be an option. Commentary is usually included with results.

### List of Tests

**Full Thyroid Panel, to include as many of these as possible:**

- TSH (Thyroid Stimulating hormone)
- Free T3
- Free T4
- Reverse T3 (difficult to obtain in the UK)
- Thyroid Peroxidase Antibodies (TPOAB)
- Thyroglobulin Antibodies (TGAB)

## Vitamins and Minerals:

- Vitamin D3
- B12
- Folate/Folic acid
- Iron, Ferritin
- Magnesium
- RBC Potassium
- Zinc
- Iodine

## Adrenals:

- 24-Hour Saliva Adrenal Test:

Taking a saliva sample at 8am, midday, 4-5pm, 11pm-midnight. Tests for Cortisol and DHEA.

## Sex Hormone Testing (for: fertility, sex hormone imbalances such as oestrogen dominance, PCOS)

- Oestrogen, Oestradiol
- Progesterone
- Testosterone
- LH
- FSH
- Prolactin

Always work with a medical professional when evaluating and re-evaluating your thyroid hormone levels, keeping in mind your symptoms and overall health as well.

**Places You Can Order Tests**

Please note that any services included in this list are not necessarily endorsed or recommended by myself. This list is kept up to date on my website, so know that you can check this online too, for any new testing companies I have become aware of.

In alphabetical order:

**All of Europe**

TrueHealthLabs
LetsGetChecked

**Arab United Emirates**

LetsGetChecked

**Australia**

NutriPath
i-Screen

**Canada**

LetsGetChecked
TrueHealthLabs

**Germany**

Medivere Diagnostics

**Netherlands**

Prohealth
Yours Healthcare

**Sweden**

HormonHarmoni.se

**Switzerland**

Ortho-Analytic

**UK**

| | |
|---|---|
| Medichecks | www.privatebloodtests.co.uk |
| LetsGetChecked | www.privatebloodtests.com |
| TrueHealthLabs | www.bloodtestslondon.com |
| Genova | Thriva |
| Blue Horizon Medicals | Smart Nutrition |

**USA**

| | |
|---|---|
| Direct Labs | True Health Labs |
| LetsGetChecked | Private MD labs |
| My Med Lab | ZRT |

# Further Sources of Information

*"Thyroid disease, you've messed with the wrong person." -*
*Rachel Hill, The Invisible Hypothyroidism*

The Invisible Hypothyroidism isn't the only source of information out there for thyroid patients. Heck, before I started my advocacy work I read up about my new diagnosis and what it meant, on what must have been *hundreds* of websites and articles. And in countless books.

However, filtering websites and books can be daunting, so I've summed up a list of places below. Those mentioned below are not necessarily endorsed by myself and I cannot control the content or opinions expressed on external websites. They are listed for you to explore.

Please also consider leaving an online review of this book, *Be Your Own Thyroid Advocate*, so that other thyroid patients know if it will help them in their own thyroid journeys. Amazon and Goodreads are popular places to do this.

You can also find more of my work, get in touch with me and join the thyroid community on:

- TheInvisibleHypothyroidism.com
- My Facebook Page:
  Search 'The Invisible Hypothyroidism'
- Instagram: @theinvisiblehypothyroidism
- Twitter: @invisible_hypo
- Pinterest: Search 'The Invisible Hypothyroidism'
- My Facebook Group: Search 'Thyroid Family'

- My Newsletter:
  newsletter.TheInvisibleHypothyroidism.com
- Thoughtful Thyroid courses: ThoughtfulThyroid.com

## *Websites*

In alphabetical order:

### Dr Jolene Brighten

Dr. Brighten is a women's health expert, coining the term 'Post Birth Control Syndrome', and sees many thyroid patients in her day to day practise in clinic. Her articles and book are down to Earth, relatable and refreshing. She's a wealth of information on women's health and hormones.

### Dr Nikolas Hedberg

Dr Nikolas Hedberg is a well-respected and praised functional medicine practitioner and Chiropractor. With lots of great articles, blogs and even podcasts on his website, there is lots to explore.

### Holtorf Medical Group

The Holtorf Medical Group specialises in optimising quality of life and being medical detectives to uncover the underlying cause of symptoms, rather than just prescribing medications to cover-up the symptoms. Therefore, their website showcases this level of knowledge with scientifically backed up articles which are shared often across social media sites.

## Hypothyroid Mom

Dana at Hypothyroid Mom went through a traumatic experience because doctors failed to monitor her hypothyroidism correctly, resulting in her losing her unborn child. So, she began blogging and advocating in pursuit of changing thyroid treatment and subsequently, lives. She covers all sorts in the articles on her site, taking a functional medicine viewpoint, often featuring doctors as content providers.

## Mary Shomon: Thyroid Patient Advocate

Mary Shomon has a very popular Facebook page and writes for various websites. She's an advocate for both underactive and overactive thyroid patients.

## Recovering With T3

Paul Robinson at Recovering with T3 created the Circadian T3 Method (CT3M), for those who do not feel better on T4-only medication such as Levothyroxine and wish to use T3 medication. His work can be found on his website Recovering with T3, as well as in his books.

## Stop The Thyroid Madness

STTM focus mainly on the power of Natural Desiccated Thyroid for the treatment of hypothyroidism and is built on patient experiences, encouraging thyroid patients to share their stories and learn from one another. I credit STTM with my confidence in switching from Levothyroxine to NDT, which has made a huge difference to my quality of life.

## The Butterfly Effect Blog

The Butterfly Effect Blog is a health and wellness website dedicated to providing research and patient-to-patient advice on healing and dealing with chronic illness. It is created by Victoria, who has Hashimoto's.

## The National Academy of Hypothyroidism

The NAH is a non-profit, multidisciplinary medical society dedicated to the dissemination of new information on the diagnosis and treatment of hypothyroidism, mainly in the USA. It is run by a group of thyroidologists, headed by Kent Holtorf M.D., David Brownstein, M.D., Denis Wilson, M.D., Michael Freidman, N.D., and Mary Shomon. Articles and blogs on all things thyroid are written in a format that is easy to understand and digest.

## Thoughtful Thyroid

Thoughtful Thyroid was created by myself and Nadha Hassen from Thyroid Transitions. We have come together to bring a thoughtful, mindful approach to healing from thyroid disease by empowering fellow thyroid patients via online courses that enable learning, understanding, good health and wellness.

## ThyroidChange

ThyroidChange is an organisation that seeks to improve the diagnosis and treatment of thyroid conditions. They are a grass-roots movement for better thyroid care.

Thyroid Change have a website full of useful articles written by doctors.

## Thyroid Nation

Thyroid Nation focuses on uplifting readers with positive articles and stories that present information learnt from personal experiences. A lot of the articles are also based around lifestyle changes and factors that can greatly improve thyroid health.

## Thyroid Patient Advocacy

A UK charity, TPA is an independent organisation that also work towards establishing better diagnosis and treatment of hypothyroidism in patients. Dr Barry Durrant-Peatfield is a Trustee and Dr Kent Holtorf a Medical Adviser. There are countless hugely informative articles written by various doctors and healthcare professionals on the site, with information for both patients *and* doctors.

## Thyroid Pharmacist, Izabella Wentz

Izabella Wentz is a well-respected pharmacist who also developed Hashimoto's. Through her own determination and knowledge as a medical professional, she has managed to reverse her Hashimoto's by implementing lifestyle and diet changes.

### Thyroid Refresh

Thyroid Refresh is an online platform that makes living a thyroid healthy lifestyle into a game. Thyroid30 is a 30-day wellness adventure that focuses on living a healthier thyroid lifestyle.

### Thyroid Transitions

Nadha at Thyroid Transitions was diagnosed with thyroid cancer and subsequently became hypothyroid after having her thyroid gland removed. Posts and information on this website promote a more mindful and conscious way of living, encouraging you to thrive with thyroid disease.

### Tired Thyroid

Tired Thyroid was created by Barbara Lougheed, a thyroid patient who was left hypothyroid after radioactive iodine treatment for Graves' hyperthyroidism. Her goal is to educate people about the fallacies that exist about thyroid treatments.

### Thyroid UK

Thyroid UK are a Thyroid Charity in the United Kingdom. They work on improving the diagnosis and treatment of thyroid disease and are often at the front of campaigns and studies.

## *Books*

Here are some books that I've found particularly helpful in my own thyroid health journey. However, I know first-hand that investing in thyroid books can be expensive, so it's also worth knowing that I've reviewed many of them and will continue to do so, on my website TheInvisibleHypothyroidism.com, so you can get a good idea of whether certain books would be beneficial to you, before spending your hard-earned cash.

In alphabetical order:

**Adrenal Fatigue: The 21st Century Stress Syndrome** by James L. Wilson, N.D, D.C, Ph.D

**Beyond The Pill** by Dr Jolene Brighten

**Diagnosis and Management of Hypothyroidism** by Gordon R B Skinner, MD, DSc, FRCPath, FRCOG

**Hashimoto's Thyroiditis: Lifestyle Interventions for Finding and Treating the Root Cause** by Izabella Wentz PharmD

**Forties on Fire** by Kathryn Kos

**Stop The Thyroid Madness: A Patient Revolution Against Decades of Inferior Thyroid Treatment** by Janie A. Bowthorpe, M.Ed

**Tears Behind Closed Doors** by Diana Holmes

**The 30-Minute Thyroid Cookbook: 125 Healing Recipes for Hypothyroidism and Hashimoto's** by Emily Kyle MS, RDN, CDN, CLT and Rachel Hill

**The End of Chronic Fatigue** by Zana Carver Ph.D and Gina Heath INHC

**The Hormone Cure** by Sara Gottfried, MD

**The Thyroid Hormone Breakthrough** by Mary J. Shomon

**What You Must Know About Hashimoto's Disease** by Brittany Henderson, MD and Allison Futterman

**Why Do I STILL Have Thyroid Symptoms? When My Lab Tests Are Normal..** by Datis Kharrazian, DHSc, DC, MS

**You, Me and Hypothyroidism: When Someone You Love Has Hypothyroidism** by Rachel Hill AKA The Invisible Hypothyroidism & Adam Gask

**Your Thyroid and how to keep it healthy.. The Great Thyroid Scandal and How to Survive it** by Dr Barry Durrant-Peatfield

# List of Thyroid (And Related) Events

*"Our voices may be small, but if we all use them together, we can be heard."* - Rachel Hill, The Invisible Hypothyroidism

What I thought would be a good addition to this book was a list of events held around the world that are good for recognising thyroid disease and raising awareness of it. Add these to your calendar if you wish to be reminded. I take part in these every year.

In month order:

**Thyroid Awareness Month**

Always held in January.

**Autoimmune Disease Awareness Month**

Always held in March.

**International Women's Day**

Always held on 8th March.

Hashimoto's and hypothyroidism are predominantly female health conditions and the issues around many women going undiagnosed or undertreated for so long has been called a 'feminist issue'. Using this annual awareness day can be great for urging other women to become more aware of thyroid disease so they're diagnosed sooner.

**International Thyroid Awareness Week**

Always held in May.

**World Thyroid Day**

Always held on 25th May.

**World Head and Neck Cancer Day**

It was on the 27th July in 2018 and I suspect a similar day in future years. This is relevant due to Thyroid Cancer being located in the neck. Thyroid cancer often leads to hypothyroidism.

**Thyroid Cancer Awareness Month**

Always held in September. Again, many thyroid cancer survivors go on to be hypothyroidism patients.

**Pregnancy and Infant Loss Awareness Month**

Always held in October. Having a thyroid condition puts you at a higher risk for losing an unborn child.

**World Mental Health Day**

Always held on 10th October, we also know that mental health conditions often come hand in hand with thyroid disease.

# Index

# References

[1] Gharib H, 2014, *The Endocrine Society Journals, Section Introduction: Emergent Management of Thyroid Disorders*, viewed 14th November 2018
<http://press.endocrine.org/doi/abs/10.1210/EME.978193670 4811.part4>

[2] Amino N, 1988, *Autoimmunity and hypothyroidism,* viewed 14th November 2018
<https://www.ncbi.nlm.nih.gov/pubmed/3066320>

[3] Viewed 14th November 2018
<https://butyoudontlooksick.com/articles/written-by-christine/the-spoon-theory/>

[4] Viewed 14th November 2018
<https://drknews.com/unraveling-thyroid-antibodies/>

[5] Viewed 14th November 2018
<https://www.theinvisiblehypothyroidism.com/take-back-control-order-your-own-thyroid-tests/>

[6] Gierach M1, Gierach J, Skowrońska A, Rutkowska E, Spychalska M, Pujanek M, Junik R, 2012, *Hashimoto's thyroiditis and carbohydrate metabolism disorders in patients hospitalised in the Department of Endocrinology and Diabetology of Ludwik Rydygier Collegium Medicum in Bydgoszcz between 2001 and 2010,* viewed 14th November 2018,
<https://www.ncbi.nlm.nih.gov/pubmed/22378092>

249

[7] Viewed 14th November 2018
<http://www.btf-thyroid.org/information/leaflets/42-congenital-hypothyroidism-guide>

[8] Hardy O, Worley G, Lee M, Chaing S, Mackey J, Crissman B, Kishnani P, 2004, *Hypothyroidism in Down Syndrome: Screening Guidelines and Testing Methodology,* viewed 14th November 2018, <https://www.ncbi.nlm.nih.gov/pmc/articles/PMC2683266/>

[9] Viewed 14th November 2014
<https://stopthethyroidmadness.com/pooling/>

[10] Viewed 26th May 2019, National Academy of Clinical Biochemistry 2002, *Laboratory Medicine Practice Guidelines: Laboratory Support for the Diagnosis and Monitoring of Thyroid Disease.*

[11] Views 26th May 2019, Hollowell, J.G., Staehling, N.W., Flanders, W.D., Hannon, W.H., Gunter, E.W., Spencer, C.A., Braverman, L.E. *Serum TSH, T4, and thyroid antibodies in the United States population (1988 to 1994): National Health and Nutrition Examination Survey (NHANES III).*

[12] Viewed 26th May 2019, Pages 8 and 12
<https://www.sps.nhs.uk/wp-content/uploads/2018/11/RMOC-Liothyronine-Guidance-v2.0-final-1.pdf>

[13] Viewed 26th May 2019, Larisch , Midgley JEM, Dietrich JW, Hoermann R., 2018,*Symptomatic Relief is Related to Serum Free Triiodothyronine Concentrations during Follow-up in Levothyroxine-Treated Patients with Differentiated Thyroid Cancer,*
<https://www.ncbi.nlm.nih.gov/pubmed/29396968>

[14] Viewed 14th November 2018
<https://www.thyroidmanager.org/chapter/adult-hypothyroidism/#toc-9-8-1-pharmacology-of-thyroid-hormone-replacement-preparations1>

[15] Nair R, Mahadevan S, Muralidharan R, Madhavan S, 2014, *Does fasting or postprandial state affect thyroid function testing?*, viewed 14th November 2018
<https://www.ncbi.nlm.nih.gov/pmc/articles/PMC4171896/>

[16] Viewed 14th November 2018
<http://www.schizophrenia.com/sznews/archives/004348.html#>

[17] Viewed 14th November 2018
<https://www.theinvisiblehypothyroidism.com/if-ndt-is-so-good-why-wont-most-doctors-prescribe-it/>

[18] Skelin M, Lucijanić T, Amidžić Klarić D, Rešić A, Bakula M, Liberati-Čizmek AM, Gharib H, Rahelić H, 2017, *Factors Affecting Gastrointestinal Absorption of Levothyroxine: A Review,* viewed 14th November 2018,
<https://www.ncbi.nlm.nih.gov/pubmed/28153426>

[19] Bach-Huynh TG, Nayak B, Loh J, Soldin S, Jonklaas J, 2009, *Timing of levothyroxine administration affects serum thyrotropin concentration,* viewed 14th November 2018,
<https://www.ncbi.nlm.nih.gov/pubmed/19584184>

[20] Stratakis CA, Chrousos GP, 1995, *Neuroendocrinology and pathophysiology of the stress system,* viewed 14th November 2018,
<https://www.ncbi.nlm.nih.gov/pubmed/8597390>

[21] Viewed 14th November 2018
<https://chriskresser.com/the-thyroid-gut-connection/>

[22] Peters S. L, Biesiekierski R, Yelland G. W, Muir J. G, Gibson P. R, 2014, *Randomised clinical trial: gluten may cause depression in subjects with non-coeliac gluten sensitivity – an exploratory clinical study,* viewed 14th November 2018,
<https://onlinelibrary.wiley.com/doi/abs/10.1111/apt.12730>

[23] Hadjivassiliou M, Sanders DS, Grünewald RA, Woodroofe N, Boscolo S, Aeschlimann D, 2010, *Gluten sensitivity: from gut to brain,* viewed 14th November 2018,
<https://www.ncbi.nlm.nih.gov/pubmed/20170845>

[24] Sategna-Guidetti C. Volta U, Ciacci C, Usai P, Carlino A, De Franceschi L, Camera A, Pelli A, Brossa C, 2001, *Prevalence of thyroid disorders in untreated adult celiac disease patients and effect of gluten withdrawal: an Italian multicenter study.* Viewed 28th May 2019
<https://www.ncbi.nlm.nih.gov/pubmed/11280546>

[25] Viewed 28th May 2019
<https://profile.thieme.de/HTML/sso/ejournals/login.htm?rd eLocaleAttr=en&type=default&subsidiary=www.thieme-connect.de&hook_url=https%3A%2F%2Fwww.thieme-connect.de%2Fproducts%2Fejournals%2Fpdf%2F10.1055%2Fa -0653-7108.pdf>

[26] Viewed 14th November 2018
<https://www.webmd.com/rheumatoid-arthritis/rheumatoid-arthritis-diet>

[27] Viewed 14th November 2018
<http://www.arthritistoday.org/what-you-can-do/eating-well/arthritis-diet/gluten-free-diet.php>

[28] Gärtner R, Gasnier BC, Dietrich JW, Krebs B, Angstwurm MW, 2002, *Selenium supplementation in patients with autoimmune thyroiditis decreases thyroid peroxidase antibodies concentrations,* viewed 14th November 2018,
<https://www.ncbi.nlm.nih.gov/pubmed/11932302>

[29] Chaudhary S, Dutta D, Kumar M, Saha S, Mondal SA, Kumar A, Mukhopadhyay S, 2016, *Vitamin D supplementation reduces thyroid peroxidase antibody levels in patients with autoimmune thyroid disease: An open-labeled randomized controlled trial,* viewed 14th November 2018,
<https://www.ncbi.nlm.nih.gov/pubmed/27186560>

[30] Schuder SE, 2005, *Stress-induced hypocortisolemia diagnosed as psychiatric disorders responsive to hydrocortisone replacement,* viewed 14th November 2018,
<https://www.ncbi.nlm.nih.gov/pubmed/16399913>

[31] Viewed 14th November 2018
<http://www.thyroiduk.org.uk/tuk/campaigns/Patient-Expereince-Survey.html>

[32] Kupka RW, Nolen WA, Post RM, McElroy SL, Altshuler LL, Denicoff KD, Frye MA, Keck PE Jr, Leverich GS, Rush AJ, Suppes T, Pollio C, Drexhage HA, 2002, *High rate of autoimmune thyroiditis in bipolar disorder: lack of association with lithium exposure,* viewed 14th November 2018,
<https://www.ncbi.nlm.nih.gov/pubmed/11958781/>

[33] Viewed 14th November 2018
<http://mythyroid.com/thyroidnodules.html>

[34] Viewed 24th November 2019
<https://www.doctorslounge.com/index.php/news/hd/668
46/>

[35] Udovcic M, Herrera Pena R, Patham B, Tabatabai L,
Kansara A, 2017, *Hypothyroidism and the Heart,* viewed 14th
November 2018,
<https://www.ncbi.nlm.nih.gov/pmc/articles/PMC5512679/>

[36] van der Heyden JT, Docter R, van Toor H, Wilson JH,
Hennemann G, Krenning EP, 1986, *Effects of caloric deprivation
on thyroid hormone tissue uptake and generation of low-T3 syndrome,*
viewed 14th November 2018,
<https://www.ncbi.nlm.nih.gov/pubmed/3740255/>

[37] Tan Z, Beiser A, Vasan R, Au R, Auerbach S, Kiel D, Wolf
P, Seshadri S, 2008, *Thyroid Function and the Risk of Alzheimer's
Disease: The Framingham Study,* viewed 14th November 2018,
<https://www.ncbi.nlm.nih.gov/pmc/articles/PMC2694610/>

[38] Viewed 14th November 2018
<https://www.theinvisiblehypothyroidism.com/why-you-
should-tell-your-doctor-youre-on-ndt/>

[39] Viewed 14th November 2018
<https://www.theinvisiblehypothyroidism.com/letter-to-my-
doctor-about-ndt/>

# Also by The Author

## *You, Me and Hypothyroidism: When Someone You Love Has Hypothyroidism*

The first resource for friends, family and other loved ones of thyroid patients, this book is a comprehensive and much-needed tool which compiles all the information you need in order to ensure your relationship doesn't suffer at the hands of this 'invisible illness'.

Included in *You, Me and Hypothyroidism*:

- Easy to understand information on what hypothyroidism is and how it affects your spouse, friend or family member
- Ways in which you can best support the person you know with hypothyroidism to get them back to good health
- Information and practical advice on fertility issues, mental health, changes in sex drive, managing social events, dietary changes, housework and more, when your loved one has hypothyroidism
- A list of resources (websites, books) for further reading

Although hypothyroidism can certainly feel like an unwelcome third wheel in a relationship, it needn't be forever. Learn not only how to overcome this change to both of your lives, but also how it can instead **strengthen** your relationship.

36926273R00152